HOW TO LIVE TO BE 100

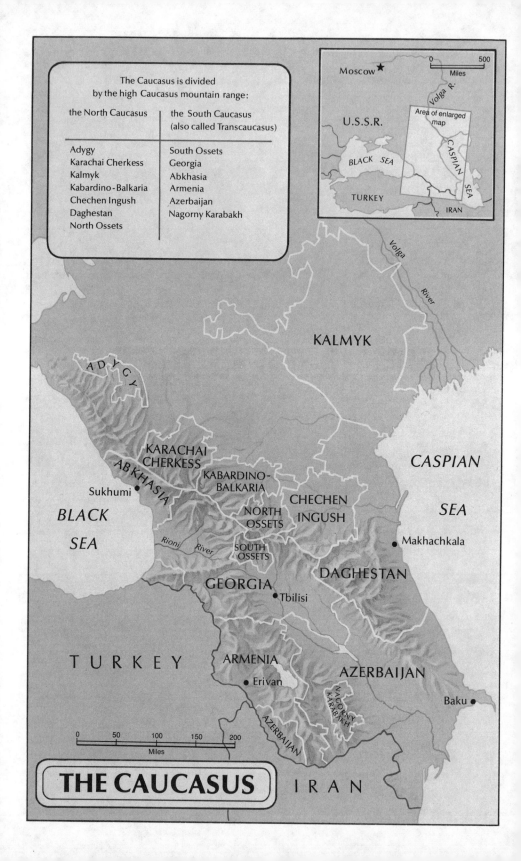

The Caucasus is divided
by the high Caucasus mountain range:

the North Caucasus	the South Caucasus (also called Transcaucasus)
Adygy	South Ossets
Karachai Cherkess	Georgia
Kalmyk	Abkhasia
Kabardino-Balkaria	Armenia
Chechen Ingush	Azerbaijan
Daghestan	Nagorny Karabakh
North Ossets	

Moscow ★

U.S.S.R.

Volga R.

Area of enlarged map

0   500
Miles

BLACK   SEA

CASPIAN   SEA

TURKEY

IRAN

Volga

River

KALMYK

ADYGY

KARACHAI CHERKESS

ABKHASIA

KABARDINO-BALKARIA

Sukhumi

NORTH OSSETS

CHECHEN INGUSH

CASPIAN

SEA

Makhachkala

BLACK

SEA

Rioni   River

SOUTH OSSETS

DAGHESTAN

GEORGIA

Tbilisi

TURKEY

ARMENIA

Erivan

AZERBAIJAN

NAGORNY KARABAKH

Baku

AZERBAIJAN

0   50   100   150   200
Miles

THE CAUCASUS

IRAN

SULA BENET

HOW TO LIVE TO BE

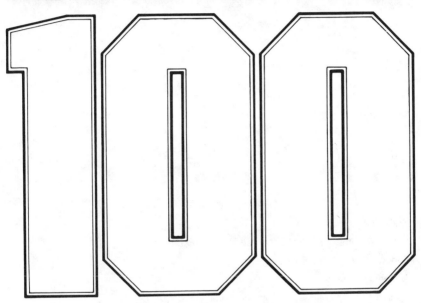

THE LIFE-STYLE OF THE PEOPLE OF THE CAUCASUS

THE DIAL PRESS   1976   NEW YORK

A portion of this book first appeared in *Catholic Digest*.

Manufactured in the United States of America

Second printing 1976

Library of Congress Cataloging in Publication Data

Benet, Sula.
    How to live to be 100.

    Bibliography: p.
    Includes index.
    1. Longevity. 2. Caucasus—Social life and customs.
I. Title. II. Title: The life-style of the people
of the Caucasus.
QP85.B45   612.6′8   75–40471
ISBN 0–8037–3834–X

To the Memory of my Dear Friend
ALFRED QUITTNER

CONTENTS

Photographs following page 48

ACKNOWLEDGMENTS

In the summer of 1970 I was invited by the Ethnographic Institute of the Moscow Academy of Sciences to do field work in the Caucasus. Since then I made frequent trips to cities, towns, and villages in the Caucasus ranging in length from six weeks to four months in the period from June 1970 to April 1975. The field work provided me with a unique opportunity to work in the area of greatest known concentration of longevous people and the area where people attain the oldest ages yet recorded for man. During my research trips I visited Abkhasia, Armenia, Azerbaijan, Georgia, Kabardino-Balkaria, Karachaiev, and North and South Ossetia. Whenever possible, I interviewed, observed, collected biographies and photographed the long-living people with their families.

The director of the Ethnographic Institute of the Moscow Academy, Academician Julian Bromley, took great interest in my work and I am indebted to him and to the members of the Caucasian Division of the Institute for their unfailing hospitality and help. I worked closely with the members of the Caucasian Division of the Ethnographical Institute. Most especially, I thank Drs. Valentin Gardanov, Jaroslava Smirnova, Galina Sergeieva, Ala Ter-Sarkisiants, and Natalia Volkova. They were all extremely generous in sharing with me their field notes and discussing interesting correlations.

In Tbilisi, Georgia, I was privileged to work with Professor Grigori A. Pitskhelauri, head of the Gerontological Institute. He is widely known in the Soviet Union for his important gerontological research in the Caucasus. He provided me with the names of longevous people in the various villages I visited and made his research available to me.

After I arrived in New York, Dr. Natalia Volkova and Dr. Ala Ter-Sarkisiants, with the permission of the Moscow Academy of Sciences, sent me a large number of photographs of very old people along with their ages and brief biographical sketches. As is the custom in the Soviet Union, all this material was accompanied by an affidavit testifying to its validity.

I am especially grateful to Professor Makhty Sultanov, a physician specializing in gerontology, for sharing with me his personal experiences and observations on the long-living people of Azerbaijan.

In Kiev the head of the Institute of Gerontology, Academician Professor D. F. Chebotarev and Dr. N. N. Sachuk, Head of the Laboratory of Demography were extremely generous in permitting me to examine their data and in inviting me to visit the Institute's Laboratory of Nutrition and Hygiene.

I am deeply grateful to Dr. Vera Rubin, Director of the Research Institute for the Study of Man, New York, for making available to me the facilities of the Institute which enabled me to complete the manuscript. I am also indebted to her for her continuing support, advice, and warm friendship which saw me through some very difficult times.

I would like to thank my friend Dr. Flora Kaplan for her critical comments on the manuscript and for editing some passages of poetry.

To Mr. Victor Geduldick, many thanks for critically reading the chapter on folk medicine. His expert pharmaceutical knowledge was most helpful.

I would like to thank Professor Harvey Pitkin for many fruitful consultations, especially in the field of Caucasian linguistics.

Mrs. Eugenie Robinson shared helpful discussions of Caucasian cuisine for which I am very thankful.

Many Russian articles and documents were ably translated for me by Mr. Michal Chusid.

My warm thanks to Joyce Engelson, executive editor at The Dial Press, whose idea it was for me to write this book, for her continued encouragement and advice.

My three last trips to the Caucasus were made possible by grants from the Faculty Research Award Program of the City University of New York, the Research Institute for the Study of Man and from the Ford Foundation. Without their help, these trips would have not been possible.

HOW TO LIVE TO BE 100

The Old Mountaineers

High in the mountains, they live,
Perhaps since the Prophet, perhaps—God knows!
Higher than all the eastern peaks
Is their esteem for personal honor.

O ancient mountaineers!
More than once
The nation acclaimed you
For your wise counsel
To the people and their rulers.

Proud are they, but not vain.
I yield the path to their horses
As I cross the mountains.
Before them,
I lower my head.

Shyly I wait, with a humble soul.
What will those who hear my verses say?
I care not for critics and their learned prose,
But for elder folk in mountain homes.

Rasul Gamzatov, a contemporary Daghestan poet
(Translated by Sula Benet)

INTRODUCTION
A VISIT WITH
THE OLDEST WOMAN
IN THE WORLD

*Adding years to life is now not as important as
adding life to years.*
—Soviet gerontologist Davydovskii

It may be difficult to believe, but I have had the pleasure of meeting and knowing a delightful woman 139 years old. Khfaf Lazuria, according to the official register of her native village of Kutol, Abkhasia, was born on October 18, 1835;—in 1974, she was perhaps the oldest woman alive. I was taken to visit Khfaf by her grandnephew, Mushni Taevich, an eminent Abkhasian poet, who drove me to Kutol early one summer morning. We found Khfaf sitting comfortably in the shade of a large tree in the courtyard of her home. The courtyard was broad and spacious, covered with smooth green grass which was kept neat and trim not with a lawn-mower, but by the numerous animals—chickens, geese, turkeys, goats, and horses—which roamed and grazed freely.

Although she had not been told of our coming, Khfaf was clearly delighted to have visitors, especially her favorite grandnephew. She kissed Mushni and immediately asked him for a cigarette. Most Abkhasians do not smoke or drink hard liquor, but this breezy lady of 139 took great pleasure in puffing on the cigarette. After warm greetings and introductions, we sat down and I began to question her. Although her Russian was limited, she understood everything I asked, and we communicated with great ease.

She was quite small. I was told that she had been taller, but had seemed to have shrunk with the years. She was about five feet tall and like most Abkhasians, slender. Her face was astonishingly smooth with few wrinkles. Her eyes were bright, curious, alive—and often full of mischief. She had a keen sense of humor and laughed easily. She responded warmly to me, kissing my cheeks as an expression of her approval. When I returned her kiss, I noticed her fresh smell, like that of a young girl. She wore a simple, blue-and-white-flowered dress made like a caftan. I could see that it had been washed

1

many times, but was spotless and neat. A white-polka-dotted cotton kerchief was wrapped around her head, and she wore pink slippers over gray stockings.

I told her I'd heard she could thread a needle without wearing glasses. She laughed. "I never had eyeglasses," she said. Would she do it for me? "Oh, yes! But we are sitting in the shade, so it must be white thread." Her great-granddaughter went into the house and brought out a needle and thread. Khfaf's agile fingers threaded the needle in just a few seconds. She held it up with a flourish. I'd prepared my camera to photograph the actual threading —an astonishing feat in itself—but she was so quick that I captured only her triumphant look as she pulled the thread through.

I asked whether her parents, too, had lived long. She said that her great-grandfather, Dzhadash, had lived to 160, and his grandson, Naruk, to 120. Her mother had also lived long. Khfaf remarked that "mother did not know how to get old," and that her first cousin, Bzhenia, lived to be 146. Khfaf had two brothers and three sisters, some of whom had died when they were "only" ninety or so, because of an epidemic. It's apparent that longevity does, indeed, run in her family. Her relatives later supported this fact.

Her smile clearly revealed some remaining teeth, but I did not have the heart to ask her how many.

I asked for a toilet and one of the young schoolgirls accompanied me to the outhouse, which was at least five city blocks away from where we were sitting. (It is customary to place the outhouses some distance from the houses.) The girl remarked, "Khfaf uses the meadow over there because there is no odor." Further along, we came to a brook with a bench placed very close to it and a pail nearby. Khfaf bathed from the pail every morning, sprinkling herself with this lovely fresh water which she preferred to tap water. Despite the fact that she had caught a cold on a chilly day the year before, she was not discouraged from this routine.

Khfaf claimed that was the only cold she ever had, that measles had been her only childhood disease, and that her health was perfect. I asked her to what she attributes her good health. She told me she eats regularly. She always carried food with her on any long trip so that she could have her meals on time. She preferred eating small quantities frequently, rather than large meals.

Khfaf urged me to accept a cigarette from her grandnephew. When I declined, she told me that she herself had not smoked at all until she was a hundred. When her work in the collective fields slowed down and she spent more time at home, she had been bored and taken up smoking: Actually, she smoked only occasionally—when someone offered her a cigarette. My guess is that, even more than smoking itself, she enjoyed the jaunty look it gave her. Indeed, she asked for a cigarette when she was about to be photographed.

She used to love horseback riding, but gave it up when she was about a hundred because there were too many cars on the road, which frightened the horses. "By the way," she joked, "how about sending me a car to drive?" She laughed and everybody there joined in the laughter.

In her younger days, in addition to working in the collective fields, she was a well-known midwife. She announced proudly that she had brought more than a hundred babies into the world.

We were expecting another guest. Mushni referred to her as the "girl Khfaf married off." To my great surprise, the "girl" turned out to be almost a century old. Khfaf looked hardly older than this woman, Adusha Lazuria, who is happily married to a relative of Khfaf's. She was seventeen when Khfaf made the match.

We spent a few hours chatting. People came and went, refreshments were served, songs were sung, and Khfaf's stepson delighted me with a demonstration of national dancing.

Then the whole household, including the stepson's daughter-in-law and her children, set up a table in the courtyard. It was a lovely day, not too hot. The usual fare appeared on the table: abista (cornmeal), chicken, boiled meat from a freshly slaughtered calf, fruit, and abundant wine for drinking and toasting. The young girls stood by with pitchers of wine ready to replenish everyone's glass. Khfaf rose and led me by the hand to the table where she seated me beside her. As the oldest, she presided over the table. To my astonishment, she had two vodkas and kept urging me to drink my wine. She was amazed when I declined the vodka.

Although I knew in a general way the intricate banquet ritual of speeches and toasting, and who must drink standing and who may remain seated, I wasn't completely clear on all the minute details. Khfaf was. She needed no prompting. I was asked to get up only once, when Khfaf made a speech in my honor.

The food was plentiful, but no one overindulged. As the hours passed in drinking, eating, and talking, Khfaf showed no sign of fatigue. I, on the other hand, beginning to feel a bit tired, absentmindedly lowered my corn-on-the-cob to my lap. Suddenly I felt something and looked down to see two chickens boldly pecking away at my corn!

What struck me most about Khfaf and about all the long-lived people I was to come to know so well in the many regions of the Caucasus was the

3

fullness of their humanity. Khfaf was interested in everything and thoroughly feminine, wearing silver rings on both hands, and examining my jewelry. She noticed a bit of lace on my petticoat and wanted to see more of it. She was a striking contrast to the "old" people in our own country, who have so often given up on life in their sixties. The idea that she should cease to have interests, desires, or feelings because she had reached a certain age would have been incomprehensible to her, or laughable.

Khfaf claimed that in her youth she never met an Abkhasian who could read or write. She herself remained illiterate, although she was fully aware that today things are very different and that everyone goes to school. Her grandnephew is a fine poet who translated Pushkin's *Eugene Onegin* into Abkhasian. She did not know Pushkin, but she understood what poetry is because she knew Abkhasian folksongs and ballads.

It is awesome to think of how much history her life-span embraced. In 1853, during the Crimean War, Khfaf was a young girl with thick braids who was taken away from Abkhasia in a Turkish boat. She did not return to her homeland until ten years later.

She married at the age of forty and gave birth to a son, but soon lost both son and husband. At fifty she married a Christian and was baptized; she was born a Muslim. Khfaf was a firm believer in marriage. Her fourth and last marriage took place in 1944 when she was 108. Recently Khfaf, concerned that her granddaughter-in-law's brother was still a bachelor, told him that it was silly not to be married and that if she had an offer she would most certainly marry again!

She was eighty-five years old in 1921 when Soviet power was established in Abkhasia. She helped to organize the first collective farm. When a new crop, tea, was introduced on the collective, she became a member of the first "tea brigade." In 1940 she traveled to Moscow for the first All-Union Agricultural Exhibition. At that time she was already 104 years old.

At the age of 128 she continued to work. During tea-harvesting time she could gather as much as twenty-five kilos a day. Her quickness and skill served as a model to other workers who learned from her how to do the job more easily.

In the Soviet village register of Kutol, under the number 469, Khfaf is listed as the head of the household although she was illiterate and extremely old. Living in Khfaf's compound, besides her stepson Tarkuk, a widower, are his youngest son, thirty-three, his wife, and their two children. The son works as a teacher at the collective.

Everyone respected and liked Khfaf. She played with the great-grandchildren, swept the large courtyard daily, took complete care of a good-size vegetable garden, and saw to all of her own needs, including her own laundry. The great respect given to old people precludes depriving them of any activity they choose to take part in. It is assumed that people of any age may participate fully in the life of the household—its duties and its pleasures.

Khfaf was not unique in the Caucasus, or even an oddity. Although the marvel of her longevity and vigor is enough in itself to delight and interest us, she was a relatively common phenomenon among the people of her region.

One day a friend called me, "Turn on your TV," said she. "Khfaf Lazuria is on." I rushed to the set but saw only the last part of Khfaf's one-hundred-fortieth birthday celebration. A delegation from Moscow had come with good wishes for Khfaf and TV cameras were there to film the occasion. Khfaf was asked to dance. She obliged. Shifting her cane from right hand to left, she alternately waved her arms as the style of the dance required. I don't think she really needed the cane to support herself. But a cane is a sign of respectability and dignity. After ninety, no one would think of being without a cane although for some it is more of a nuisance than a help.

On a very cold day in autumn, Khfaf Lazuria, faithful to her custom, took her daily bath in the mountain stream. The next day she had a fever, and finally had to admit that she did not feel well. After two weeks, she asked her family to accompany her to the family cemetery which was about a city block away. She wished to select her burial place. She pointed to the grave of her husband. "There," she said, "I have no right to be buried because I was his second wife and I will not see him in the next world. His first wife is buried next to him and she will be with him in the next world. I would like to be buried here. . . ." and she pointed to a place a bit higher—a lovely spot overlooking a meadow filled with flowers. She died on February 14, 1975.

I learned of her death from television, radio, and press reports. A month later I was able to visit her family. How different it was from my visit of a few months before. The family was subdued and quiet in her absence, and the house seemed bare and empty without her.

Her granddaughter-in-law took me to the cemetery. We had to climb a rather high fence in order to get there and I wondered silently how Khfaf had managed it. Before the fence, the young woman smiled, observing my hesitation. "Khfaf," she said, "used to come this way twice a day, saying that it would soon be her next home." Well, I am a pretty agile climber, with good balance, and I found that fence rather difficult to manage. And Khfaf did it twice a day every day before she died!

A small wooden structure resembling a hut covered the grave, but it was open enough for me to see inside. There, a small table held a pitcher of water with a glass, and close by lay a package of cigarettes and matches, for Khfaf's use. It was strange to observe this pagan tradition, which the family felt was completely fitting, harmoniously merged with Christian burial rites. Back at the house, I was shown a room upstairs where a table had been prepared, displaying photographs of Khfaf at various stages of her life, lit by a candle like a shrine.

My involvement in the study of Khfaf and her people has its own history, with roots that reach deep into my early memories. As a child, I lived in Warsaw, Poland. My father made frequent business trips to the Caucasus and my mother often went there to "take the waters." They returned with colorful stories of the wonderful people with whom they had become friends in that land of towering mountains, plunging ravines, and remote villages. They promised to take me there someday and I yearned to go, but it was not to be—then.

My imagination had been firmly captured and my interest persisted, nonetheless. I read everything I could find in history and fiction about the land and its people. And the literature was abundant. Despite the fierce conflict between Russia and those Caucasians who resisted annexation, Russian writers of the second half of the nineteenth century celebrated the Caucasus lyrically. Pushkin, Lermontov, and Tolstoy found these proud people a source of inspiration.

Many years later, when I was grown and living on another continent, many miles from those enchanted mountains, the childhood dream curiously became a reality. It happened by chance and not by my design. As a professor of anthropology at Hunter College in New York, I had been asked to translate and edit for Doubleday & Co. an ethnographic study of a small Russian village. The study had been published originally by the Ethnographic Institute of the Academy of Science in Moscow. One fine spring day in 1970, after my translation had been published, I received a cable from the Academy officially inviting me to do ethnographic field work in Abkhasia. I hardly remembered where it was, except that it was in the Caucasus, and that was all I needed. Without stopping even to look at a map, I went straight to the telegraph office and sent a return cable to the Academy: "Thank you. Coming."

There was something so utterly right and fitting about such a study. I could hardly believe my good fortune. To be able to visit the land of my childhood fantasies, not as a tourist, but doing my chosen life work—as an anthropologist, to observe and record the daily lives of its people, and to share what I found there with others—what luck! It was as if things had come full circle for me and I could hardly wait for the school term to end so that I could get started. The time was spent in learning all I could about the people to whom I was going—and whom I had visited so many times in my imagination.

During that field trip, in which I conducted studies on the early collectivization of the villages, the people I interviewed kept referring me to older people who, they said, would know more than they did, since collectivization had taken place some forty years before. These old people did indeed remember the earliest times. I found myself interviewing an unusually large number of people who ranged in age from 80 to 110, all of whom were still active in village life.

They talked easily with me, answering a great number of questions, and expressed opinions on the advantages and disadvantages of a collective economy. I was especially impressed by their cheerfulness, vigor, and humor, and made many friends among them. Their lives, their work, and their important roles in the village were indeed fascinating, but beyond that, I grew increasingly interested in learning *why* they lived so long, and in such apparent health, good spirits, and productivity.

Since earliest antiquity, the Caucasian peoples have been known for their legendary longevity. Ancient Greek, Iranian, and Arabian chronicles attest amply to the existence of long-living peoples throughout the region. The latest Soviet census reported that 70 per cent of all people reaching 110 years or more live in the Caucasian republics; the remaining 30 per cent are found in all the territories of European Russia, Siberia, the Ukraine, Central Asia, and Kazakstan.

There was nothing new in the *fact* of the Caucasians' longevity. What I wanted to discover was the reason for it. I was often tempted to ask them how they got to be so old, but felt it would have been in poor taste. Sometimes, however, they themselves would volunteer the answer: "I live the right way," they would say proudly. But what was the right way?

In an effort to find answers to this complex question, I have returned six more times to the Caucacus between the summer of 1970 and the spring of 1975. Like all field work, it was not always easy, and sometimes quite difficult, especially in winter when mountain roads were icy and in some places impassable. Nestled between high-rising mountains, many villages are isolated from the outside world except for narrow paths, negotiable only in summer and only by experienced climbers. From the steep mountainsides above, the gigantic white tongues of glaciers descend almost to the edge of the villages. But it was important to see the people in all seasons, to see how they adapted their work and activities to seasonal changes.

I was fortunate to be able to speak fluent Russian, so that we could communicate directly, without translators. It is assumed outside the Soviet Union that all Caucasians are Russians. This is a misconception and, unfortunately, a widespread one. Although Russian is the official language and mandatory in the schools, and there are sizable Russian populations in many Caucasian cities, the Caucasus is a geographical area made up of many different republics and autonomous areas, such as Georgia, Azerbaijan, Abkhasia, Armenia, Daghestan, and scores of others, large and small. Each of the many groups speaks and writes its own language and keeps its own customs and traditions, although Russian is used for communication between the different republics and the central government.

The Caucasian people live not only a long time, but in health and strength. Soviet scientists have found few if any cases of the degenerative diseases which plague the United States and Russia proper, such as heart disease, arteriosclerosis, kidney stones, gall stones, coronary occlusion, and hypertension.

An Azerbaijanian gerontologist, Dr. Makhty Sultanov, observed a 117-year-old man in Kabardino-Balkaria who splits and saws logs for his hearth routinely. I was told by Said, a Caucasian ethnographer, of a man of ninety in the village of Kurchaloi, who lifted a ram by the scruff of the neck just to show that "he was still a man." This same ethnographer told of a 120-year-old man who married a woman of forty and fathered three children.

Numerous Soviet medical teams have researched, observed, and documented many similar facts. I myself saw old people in the Caucasus riding horses, weeding vigorously, swimming, presiding over feast tables, participating in all the activities of family and community life, with no signs of exhaustion or fatigue. It seemed quite natural that Makhty Tarkil, a strikingly handsome, tall Abkhasian of 104, during the banquet his family gave in my honor, frequently patted my hand, offered to give me a fine horse as a gift, and generally behaved like a courting gentleman. It was inconceivable that men or women there, no matter how old, could think of themselves as merely existing, marking time waiting for death, unloved, unwanted, and useless. These old men and women would not think of missing the village competition in horseracing.

What a contrast to our American "senior citizens" in their sixties and seventies! Here, in the richest, most technologically advanced country in the world, older people are farmed out, discarded, hidden away in hospitals, nursing "homes," artificial retirement villages, or falsely cheerful apartment compounds. To be old means to be exiled from the active life of society.

In American culture, the individual loses value as he ages. He is considered a worn-out model by his employer, an old car to be traded in. He is treated more and more like a minor by his family. Once having attained maturity, brief as it is in American society, he is automatically on the road back to infantilism. His teen-age children inform him, in increasingly less subtle ways, that he is "old-fashioned" and unable to adapt to changing conditions. He is "over thirty" and untrustworthy. As he gets older, he is treated as increasingly forgetful, irresponsible, outdated, and outdistanced, and in keeping with this treatment, he begins to conform to expectations—we react as we are treated. Responsibility is taken from him, and in the "second childhood" he is thought to be fit only for childish games, like shuffleboard. He reacts by becoming infantile, making petty demands, being ill-tempered and unreasonable. He seems to want to return to "the good old days," which really means the period when he was considered a responsible adult.

The old in America envy the young, since the young are the center of all ongoing life. The young in turn look at the old with scorn and an air of superiority, feeling that they know everything and their parents are too old and conservative to grasp the changes in the world. Tension permeates the relations between the generations—the old try to keep up with the young, just as the middle class competes with the upper class and the poor try to climb into the middle class. In a society in which people are in constant competition, as individuals and in social groups, there is little relaxation or enjoyment.

Modern society creates a higher standard of living and at the same time makes greater demands on human psychological and biological organization often disturbing or destroying the physical environment in the process. This has a double effect, both positive and negative, on longevity. While creating the objective hygienic and material conditions for the prolongation of life, it destroys traditional family structure, depriving the elderly of the emotional support of their relatives and of the feeling of being needed, thus counteracting the positive effects of the higher material standard of living.

Caucasian culture, admittedly, represents an older, more stable system, with minimal industrialization and technological change—hardly comparable structurally or economically. Nonetheless, the integrated culture of the Caucasus, where all age groups and social classes live in symbiosis and cooperation to the mutual advantage of all concerned, has much to teach modern industrial society, which for all its technology and higher material standard of living has not improved the quality of life nor met the basic social needs of humans of any age. A person, modern society has once again realized, is not infinitely plastic, but has psychological, biological, and social needs which demand attention and satisfaction. Any material or technological system which fails to take these needs into consideration is doomed to self-destruction.

Twenty-five per cent of our current 210 million population is now over the age of sixty; this represents 52.5 million people. About 8 million people are seventy-five or over. The increased longevity of our population is going to have a tremendous impact on all aspects of society. It behooves us to take a long, hard look at societies where old age is graceful, harmonious, and productive.

Since the 1930s, Soviet scientists, in local gerontological institutes, have been studying the aged of the Caucasus medically and demographically. The Institute of Gerontology in Kiev, which is the center for gerontological studies, coordinates the findings of the local institutes. I had ample opportunity to discuss longevity with scientists and medical personnel at the various centers. They were most generous in permitting me to see their unpublished research as well as their published articles. I benefited greatly from their experience, but medical research, as important as it is, could not answer the question of why we find this great concentration of longevity in the Caucasus and not, for instance, in Russia proper or in the Ukraine. Neither could medical research answer the question of how the Caucasians preserved their faculties.

The secret of their longevity, and its healthy, satisfied, vigorous quality, can best be probed by a thorough inquiry into their total environment and culture. Accordingly, this book begins with a historical background of the Caucasus region, from the time of the earliest explorations by the Greeks and Romans. Then the land and its peoples are examined, the geography, ecology, economics, occupations, family, and community structure. This background provides the setting for an observation of the people on a daily basis—their family life, hospitality, village political organization, the place of old people, recreational activities and celebrations, folk medicine, and diet. Their attitudes on work, marriage, sexuality, and aging itself will also emerge.

1
AN ANTHROPOLOGIST GOES TO THE CAUCASUS

Any anthropologist setting out to do field work is all too well aware of the problem of "objectivity," of the constant admonition to remain as "culture free" or "value free" as possible. As every first-year anthropology student learns, the cardinal principle of field work is to be objective. As a scientist observing and recording phenomena of a culture foreign and alien to one's own, one must make every effort to avoid invidious comparisons and judgmental thinking. Complete scientific detachment may or may not be possible to human beings, all of whom, to a greater or lesser degree, are bound to see the world through the prism of their own culture. We can only try.

It is clear that an integral part of any anthropologist's objectivity is a sincere effort to *perceive the culture under study as its people see it.* We must analyze and evaluate their behavior in terms of *their* motivation and cultural assumptions, not our own. It is required of the reader as well to make an effort to suspend his own culture-bound perceptions of what is "normal" or acceptable.

All of this is, of course, not simple. Among the pleasures and tribulations of the anthropologist are several common temptations against which one must be on guard, even though an occasional lapse may sometimes enrich the humanity of any study. One of these is the tendency to become protective toward the people with whom we spend so much time in the process of collecting data. There is a standard joke about the frequent use of the phrase "my tribe" at any gathering of anthropologists. However unprofessional or unscientific, it is difficult to remain icily detached from real people whom we come to know and admire, and this proprietory phrase usually reflects a genuine affection.

In my own case, given a people as attractive, energetic, and hospitable as

13

the Caucasians, the risk of overstating their positive qualities is even greater. But it is a risk worth taking, and I trust that I have been able to adhere to the mandate of objectivity insofar as that is possible.

This is not to say that there were not some cultural assumptions I found extremely difficult to deal with in a neutral manner, most notably those which have to do with women. As one who assumes a firm position on the equality of women, I was often very ill-at-ease in observing certain customs and rules of behavior which reflect women's subservience to men. For example, as a guest, I was always afforded the special privilege of sitting at the dinner table with the men, but it never ceased to cause me the greatest discomfort to remain seated while the younger women of the household stood dutifully behind our chairs. This custom, of course, prevails mostly in the rural areas, especially where Moslem tradition is the strongest.

The social dominance of the men made it difficult to evoke the women's views in interviewing, and I sought ways to circumvent this problem. For example, I found that one of the most useful—and pleasant—ways to get people chatting easily was to bring up the topic of food and recipes. Whenever conversations lagged or people seemed a bit reticent, I would talk of food; it never failed to produce a warm and informal atmosphere, with everyone eager to share what he or she knew. The men, of course, took the lead in answering my questions, assuming that it was they, rather than the women, who knew the answers to anything an important guest might ask, even in the matter of food. To avoid this, I would often ask for specific recipes, which most of the men, however expert they thought they were, rarely knew. It was a splendid way of getting into the kitchen with the women, who would then feel free to chat about all manner of things. The informality of "kitchen talk" provided me with a great deal of interesting data from the women which they would not have been able to share in the presence of the men.

There are discomforts of a physical and psychological nature present in any anthropological field work, but those I experienced in the Caucasus were minimal. There is the ever-present hardship of getting around in mountainous terrain, of climbing rocky slopes and steep pathways in order to arrive anywhere. This is certainly unaccustomed physical exertion for an urban American, used to taxis and elevators, and I huffed and puffed my way through all of it. The physical benefits, however, were quite apparent on my return, when I found that stairways that I might usually avoid were easy to climb.

The same is true of the food which, on the whole, I found quite palatable, but which occasionally was flavored with a sauce which brought tears to my eyes and left me speechless. Following their example, I ate a great deal of what they refer to as "grasses," that is, greens and edible plants which they forage for in the forest, and fruits in large quantities. This practice very definitely diminished my desire for meats and carbohydrates. Sugar was totally absent from my diet, with only an occasional bit of honey. Without any conscious effort, I lost ten pounds during the first three weeks and felt physically strong and energetic.

I also received the benefits of their excellent folk medicine one day while taking a shortcut on a wooded mountain slope with a boy of seven or eight. A sharp branch in the underbrush cut my calf and it began to bleed; the boy quickly found a blade of grass and placed it on the wound, which immediately stopped bleeding. The grass was generally known to possess this coagulative property.

My attempt in learning and considering Caucasian customs earned me many friends. To show their appreciation, on the Fourth of July, I received flowers, boxes of chocolate, and messages with best wishes written on Russian congratulation cards. My friends learned about the American holiday from my assistant and decided that it must be equivalent to the First of May in the Soviet Union.

In an effort to maintain objectivity, I purposefully limit the length of each field trip. Over the years, I noticed that my effectiveness as an observer required short, frequent trips to insure freshness of perception and sensitivity.

My linguistic facility was a great advantage in that it enabled me to record cultural nuances which often disappear or become distorted in translation.

This is an anthropological study which seeks to describe, analyze, and evaluate a life-style which has produced an unusually large number of long-living people. My goal is to provide some insights into the reasons for this longevity. Isolated examples of longevity are, of course, not unique. What makes the Caucasians unique is the very high number of healthy centenarians in their population. The percentage of longevous people far exceeds that found in Ecuador or among the Hunzas of Pakistan, for example.

The problem of aging and death is of interest to all of us, and the focus of this study is on those intrinsic factors found in Caucasian life which seem to be conducive to long life and good health. It is not my intention either to praise or to condemn the traditions, as ancient as the Bible, by which the Caucasians live. As an anthropologist, I pass no judgment on the people I study; I try to understand them.

Every society has its light and shadow, its integral whole, its own history, environment, and evolution. There are patterns of behavior and survival, however, which are universal to all humans as biological organisms. The elements of Caucasian society which are unquestionably beneficial to their physical well-being may well be useful in our own thinking about health and aging. My object, of course, is to describe and not to prescribe. Despite rituals and traditions we may reject, we can, nonetheless, learn how *they* live and attain healthy old age. We may even be able to adapt or modify some of their practices, such as diet, exercise, and emphasis on regularity of daily routine, to our own lives. It is also quite clear that the attitudes of family and community toward the elderly have a profound effect on their longevity.

There are, of course, many more nationalities and ethnic groups in the Caucasus than are discussed in the book. I have selected for study only those areas known to have exceptionally large numbers of longevous people. This selection is based on demographic data obtained from the population census of 1970 and medical records. It would be very satisfying to be able to describe every group present in the region, but I am limited first, by the size of the book, and second, by the fact that I am focusing on the question of longevity and not just ethnography.

I think it important to say that I do not presume to recommend a way of life that will insure longevity. When I contend that a specific practice is "good" for one, it means that it is good for health and longevity, *as I observed it in the Caucasus.*

Change is slow in Caucasian society. Gradual change is, indeed, taking place, but without the dramatic and disorienting upheavals occurring in most of the rest of the world. Any society with even a modicum of stability and harmony in the second half of the twentieth century may seem to be an anachronism, and therefore liable to be regarded with skepticism. Nonetheless, many ancient rituals and traditions of the Caucasus do, indeed, coexist peacefully with the demands and exigencies of the modern world. Others, of course, are disappearing. Some traditions are not only outmoded, but occasionally difficult and inconvenient, but even some of these are observed *pro forma* by both young and old, especially in rural areas.

The main reason for the endurance of tradition seems to me to lie in an extraordinary willingness on the part of both the old and the young to make concessions to each other. The young, while no longer believing in the compulsory nature of old rituals, observe some of the outmoded formalities merely out of respect for the elders and to preserve harmony, and also out of a certain pride in their own national life. The old people, although aware of the inevitable changes taking place all around them, nevertheless appreciate the observance of formal rites and rituals as symbols of the past and as an affirmation of their national identity. This is perhaps the key: throughout the historical development of this region, survival demanded strong identification with one's group. It was the only defense against the endless invasions and attacks from strangers, and against intergroup wars and blood feuds.

This group identity, which still exerts a strong influence, provides a common ground for understanding between generations and insures cultural continuity. Even the most sophisticated, city-educated young and middle-aged Caucasians manifest a desire to preserve cultural traditions in some form. There are two strong currents: one has its source in the Soviet system and its resulting ties with Moscow; the other, in a passionate drive for preservation and development of national cultural traditions. There are endless discussions in the local press as to which customs should be kept and which are harmful relics and should be discarded.

There are outward appearances of change, especially in the matter of dress. More money is being spent on clothing, especially for small children and school-age youngsters. Even the villages have not escaped the now worldwide craze for American jeans, which are considered high style. The old women continue to wear dark dresses and kerchiefs, and traditional dress still appears on the holidays.

More varieties of food are available now. In addition to vegetables, fruit, and meat grown at home, there are now factory-made sweets, cakes, and, most likely, food preservatives. Forks, knives, and napkins are now commonly used at the table, yet the ritual handwashing before and after meals is still generally practiced.

The family budget in the villages is gradually changing. People spend more money on books, newspapers, radios, and electrical appliances. One finds more furniture in the rural homes than formerly and much of it is factory-made rather than handmade. Handmade carpets on the walls are still highly prized and passed from generation to generation.

In the Caucasus, the impact of industrialization came in the form of greater accessibility of consumer goods, availibility of mass culture, and mechanization in farm work. But except in certain urbanized areas—in Baku, for example—industrialization was not the same socially disruptive process that it was in the West or even in other parts of the Soviet Union. Industrialization meant the application of modern technology to farm work, not a sudden exodus from rural areas into the cities and disruption of traditional society. Collectivization here, unlike some other areas of the Soviet Union, was not accompanied by social upheaval, but in fact was mediated through *the existing channels of traditional society*: the family and community collective. Because of the revered position the elderly enjoyed in the family and the continued role that they play in the life of the collective, respect for tradition continues to be one of the most highly prized virtues.

Industrialization has also meant an increasing flow of the intelligentsia *into* the rural habitats, rather than out of them as occurred in other industrializing areas. This factor is making a qualitative change in the social structure of the rural community. Each village has its agronomists, doctors, teachers, technicians, and librarians with college degrees. In most cases, local people who have received their education in the city return to their village and families as professionals.

All of this is contributing to a gradual shift of rural power in the conduct of village affairs from the hands of the very old (Councils of Elders) to the middle-aged and the younger members of the community, and, even more strikingly, women are now assuming rights and powers hitherto unknown to them. In general, women may now participate on an equal footing with men in the village Soviet.

I can point to many other sociologic, economic, and historic factors which seem to permit the gradual, assimilating change we see taking place in the Caucasus. This slow transformation allows the old to give way gracefully to the new. As an observer of their daily lives, it seems to me, in the final analysis, that the strongest stabilizing factor remains the relationship between parents and children.

The young people still look to their parents (and grandparents) or siblings of the same sex as models, as a frame of reference for their own behavior, and as the source of their personal identity and values. There is no need to reject values which continue to give satisfaction and sustenance to the individual, and which remain valid even in the face of modern change.

Most young people to whom I talked seem to want to grow up to have the same virtues as their parents, and praise from their parents means a great deal more than the praise of their friends. I was very much interested in the parent-peer orientation; there was no doubt in my mind of the relative weight carried by the two groups: in a choice between winning the approval of their parents or that of their peer group, especially in a matter of basic values, it is plainly the parents who win out.

Peer orientation, of course, increases when students attend universities away from home, and, in general, girls are more strongly influenced by parental values than boys.

The parents, on their part, are well aware that they must serve as models, that they must teach their children by the example of their lives rather than through lectures or empty words of advice. Love and emotional support are, by the same token, demonstrated by deeds rather than public displays of affection and verbal reassurances. It is true that to an outside observer, families appear reserved and undemonstrative, but that same observer cannot help but feel the love and respect that is manifest in almost every action of family members toward each other. This, I believe, is their greatest strength.

I truly enjoyed the work in the Caucasus and am most grateful to the people for their gracious hospitality and their openness in sharing with me the lore of their ancient culture. It is hoped that this body of information, however remote it may seem from our own way of life, will in some way contribute to our understanding of the aging process. But even more, that we may begin to view old age as an integral and valued part of each of our lives.

2
THE LAND
AND ITS PEOPLE

WHO ARE THE CAUCASIANS?

The Caucasus is a land bridge, between Asia and Europe, bordered on the west by the Black Sea and on the east by the Caspian Sea. In the north, it merges into the Russian steppes and in the south, it borders Iran and Turkey. Across this country stretches the Great Caucasian Range, with altitudes exceeding 10,000 feet. The range contains the loftiest peaks in Europe (Elbrus, the highest European mountain, is 18,468 feet; Kazbeg is 16,558 feet). The high mountains are cut by deep and narrow ravines which are difficult to approach.

There are two passes, the Darial and the Derbent, which played an important part in the history of the Caucasus. From the Northern Caucasus to Transcaucasia, the shortest route is through the Darial Ravine (Darial means "gate" in Persian). To prevent invasion, the gorge was barred with real gates of wood studded with iron. The route of the present Georgian Military Road which passes through the gorge has been used since the first century B.C. by merchants of many lands as well as the Caucasian peoples.

In the upper zone, the mountains are covered with magnificent alpine and subalpine meadows which serve as pasture for tens of thousands of cattle, sheep, and horses. Flowers of great beauty and abundance blossom on the southern slope. Below is the zone of thick woods and, still further below, excellent fruit trees and grapes. Inaccessible mountains, covered by impassable, thick woods, become lost in the clouds. Turbulent streams rush down the mountains over huge cliffs.

HISTORICAL BEGINNINGS

Since remote antiquity, the Caucasus has been an enchanted land for many peoples. For the Greeks, the Caucasian Mountains represented the mysterious edge of the world where Prometheus was bound in agony as punishment by Zeus for giving fire to humanity. It was to the Caucausus, too, that the young Greek, Phrixus, and his sister, Helle, fled on a magic golden ram, escaping from their father, King Athamas, who planned to sacrifice Phrixus to the gods. But on the journey, Helle fell off the ram and drowned in the strait which was thereafter known as Hellespont. On arriving at Colchis, which is now part of Georgia and called Kolkhida, Phrixus sacrificed the golden ram, obeying the wishes of the gods. He sheared the ram and hung the fleece in a sacred grove guarded by a fire-spewing dragon. This was the famous Golden Fleece which Jason, nephew of the king of Thessaly, was sent to bring back.

In Greek mythology, Jason's exploits and adventures and those of the heroes who accompanied him in the ship *Argo* on the voyage to Colchis are well known. They encountered great dangers and visited many lands along the coast of Asia Minor. One intriguing spot was the Caucasian home island of the Amazons, a group who later migrated to Asia Minor.

At the time of the Argonauts' expedition, which Greek chronologists placed in the thirteenth century B.C., the Colchis were ruled by King Aeëtes. Aeëtes refused to give the Golden Fleece to the Greek strangers, even though he was promised the defense of his country from the surrounding warring tribes in return. However, his beautiful daughter, Medea, fell in love with Jason at first sight. Through secret sorcery, she helped Jason obtain the Golden Fleece, thus betraying her father. Afraid of her father's anger and unable to part with Jason, she consented to sail with him to Greece. When the Argonauts fled back with the Golden Fleece, many of them were wounded, but Medea skillfully healed them with roots and herbs that she had brought with her. As in all Greek tragedies, there is no happy ending. Jason fell in love with a Greek princess, and Medea in desperation killed her own children because they had been begotten by Jason.

Two of the Argonauts, twin brothers, are credited with founding the city of Dioscuria, presently Sukhumi, the capital of Abkhasia, on the shore of the Black Sea.

The students of the University of Tbilisi, the Georgian capital, decided to duplicate the journey made by the Argonauts. In 1974, they built a ship, called it the *Argo,* and sailed to Greece, visiting all the places described in Homer's *Odyssey.*

In his first-century geography, Strabon, the Greek geographer, said about the Colchis: "There are untold riches of gold, silver, and iron in their land." It seems quite possible that the Argonauts' expedition was undertaken not for the Golden Fleece but for the remarkable Colchis bronze, copper, wine, and honey.

A Roman, Pliny the Elder, who died in 79 A.D., wrote about Dioscuria: "Now these cities are neglected, but in the past, 300 tribes, speaking different languages, converged on the city and our Romans conducted their business with the help of 130 translators."

On the Caucasian shores of the Black Sea the most distant Greek colonies were founded, later to be replaced by Roman settlements and, in the Middle Ages, by Italian. Over the centuries, there were many invaders: the Roman legions, the Persian Shakhs, the Tatar Mongolian Khans. They all attempted to conquer the Caucasus, lured by its strategic position and by its natural wealth. Now from far corners of the world scientists and laymen come to the Caucasus, all seeking the magic "key" to the well-known longevity of the Caucasian peoples.

There are parallels and mutual borrowings between early Greeks and Caucasians in epic literature, mythology, and ethnobotany. For example, the great culture hero of Greek mythology, Prometheus, appears in the same role of benefactor to humanity, who suffered punishment for his important gift to his people. He is called Amirani in Georgian, Abrskil in Abkhasian, Amran in Ossetian, and Mkher in Armenian. But the theme is always the same.

A marble grave plate, unmistakably Greek, attests to the contact between the Greeks and the Caucasians. Recently found along the western edge of the Caucasus at the bottom of the Black Sea, the plate pictures two women and a boy. It is dated by archaeologists as of the fifth century B.C. and was probably imported from Greece.

FLORA AND FAUNA

A remarkable feature of the Caucasus is the continuity and persistence over long periods of time of plants, animals, human races, and human cultures. Plants long extinct in other parts of the world survive and even flourish in the Caucasus. A good illustration is the long-needle pine, growing there since the Tertiary period (at least 60 million years ago) and the groves of a unique variety of Pinus pinaster in Western Georgia.

The fauna of the Caucasus is also ancient. Here are found the Caucasian goat, chamois, Caucasian deer, roe deer, gazelle, wild boar, snow leopard, lynx, striped hyena, jackal, and other species unique to the Caucasus. Among the birds are pheasant, mountain turkey, Caucasian grouse, and swan. In the rivers and lakes are trout, salmon, carp, and sheatfish, as well as Colchis barbel, and several other species which exist nowhere else in the world.

Archaeological digs reveal the bones of many still familiar animals: cows, sheep, horses, donkeys, and dogs. These animals have been widely domesticated by people in this region for the last 5,000 years and probably even longer. It is quite possible that Transcaucasia, the southern Caucasus, was one of the earliest centers of the domestication of animals, probably before the Neolithic period. Even now, in the mountains of Armenia and other Caucasian areas, one meets with wild sheep and goats.

The Caucasian peoples developed an efficient and successful adaptation to their land. In the rocky, mountainous regions where there was little or no arable land, the basis of their livelihood and wealth was pastoralism combined with limited horticulture. In the fertile plains there was agriculture with some pastoralism. The Caucasus has great natural diversity and many microzones which have been successfully exploited by different local groups.

ETHNIC GROUPS

The Great Caucasian Range separates the Northern Caucasus from Transcaucasia. The Caucasian republics include over 200 ethnic groups, each having a separate and distinct language. The Northern Caucasus is administratively organized under the Russian Soviet Federated Socialist Republics. It includes the autonomous republics of Daghestan, North Ossetia, Kabardino-Balkar, and Chechen-Ingush; and the Karachai-Cherkess and Adygei autonomous regions.

The Transcaucasian region to the south includes the three union republics of Georgia, Azerbaijan, and Armenia. The first two encompass autonomous republics and regions: Abkhasia, Adjaria, and South Ossetia in Georgia; Nakhichevan and Nagorny-Karabach in Azerbaijan.

The ethnic groups vary considerably in size. Azerbaijan, for example, has a population of over 5 million in a territory of 53,000 square miles. Georgia, with an area of 29,000 square miles, somewhat smaller than Maine, has a population of close to 5 million. By contrast, the Archi in Daghestan occupy one village and seven neighboring farms.

There is a considerable difference between the cultures of the Northern Caucasus and Transcaucasia. The southern republics of Transcaucasia— Georgia, Armenia, and Azerbaijan—developed political states in ancient times. They have had their own written languages, literature, and a well-developed agriculture. On the other hand, until the October Revolution, the Northern Caucasus was an area populated by small national groups, each ruled by a feudal patriarchal structure. In the south, the population was relatively dense, numbering in the millions, while in the north were small ethnic pockets sometimes consisting of only a few villages.

There were a number of reasons for this difference. In the north, arable land was very scarce. In many areas of Daghestan, people bought and carried bags of soil to spread over rocks. The meager food supply yielded by limited horticulture and distant pasture sheep breeding could not support a large population. Intertribal wars and family feuds claimed many victims. Captured warriors and their families were sold by the thousands into foreign slave-holding lands, such as Turkey.

TABLE 1: Caucasian Population by Administrative Subdivision as of January 15, 1970

Northern Caucasus	
Adygei A.R.*	386,000
Karachai-Cherkess A.R.	345,000
Daghestan A.S.S.R.†	1,429,000
Kabardinian-Balkar A.S.S.R.	589,000
North Ossetian A.S.S.R.	533,000
Checheno-Ingush A.S.S.R.	1,065,000
Southern Caucasus	
Georgian S.S.R.‡	4,688,000
Abkhasian A.S.S.R.	487,000
Adjarian A.S.S.R.	310,000
South Ossetian A.R.	100,000
Azerbaijan S.S.R.	5,111,000
Nakhichevan A.S.S.R.	202,000
Nagorny-Karabakh A.R.	149,000
Armenian S.S.R.	2,493,000

*A.R. stands for Autonomous Region.
†A.S.S.R. stands for Autonomous Soviet Socialist Republic.
‡S.S.R. stands for Soviet Socialist Republic.

During the annexation of the Caucasus by the Russians in the nineteenth century, Moslems in many areas were either "encouraged" to leave or voluntarily left for Turkey hoping for freedom of religion. But after bitter disappointments, many returned. Yet some remained and the colony grew. In Turkey today there are more Abkhasians and Cherkessians than there are in the Caucasus.

Until the beginning of the process of national consolidation, the peoples of the Northern Caucasus had no cultural or political ties to unite them. The significant vestiges of communal clan society, the mountains, the patriarchal way of life, the dominance of the feudal aristocracy, civil wars, foreign invaders—all gave rise to a large number of peculiarities in the region. Customs were strictly local in character, restricted often to the area of a few ravines and sometimes to a single village. Even after the union of Northern Ossetia, Checheno-Ingushetia, Kabardino-Balkaria, and Daghestan with Russia, and even after the beginning of trade relations, the ethnic groups of these regions, in essence, remained separate nationalities.

PHYSICAL TYPES

A great variety of physical types is found in the Caucasus. This is not surprising, considering the checkered history of the area and its extraordinary ethnic diversity. The people of the area all belong to the Mediterranean type of the Caucasian race, except for some small Mongolian ethnic groups. On the whole, one may say that dark hair and eyes prevail, especially in Azerbaijan; but there is a noticeable admixture of light-eyed and blond-haired individuals in the Northern Caucasus and in Georgia. Sharply protruding noses are common. The shape of the head varies from long to extremely round. In stature, some, like most Azerbaijanians, are rather short, while others, like Daghestanians, are tall.

Archaeological findings reveal that the physical types in the Caucasus were once more closely related than they are now. Invasions and intermarriages have increased the variety of human population.

LANGUAGES

The Caucasus has been known for a long time as one of the most ethnically diverse parts of the world, with a striking variety of mutually unintelligible languages, physical types, and religious persuasions. The ancient Arabic world knew this mountainous land as "Yubel-al-Suni," or "the mountain of languages."

In the tenth century, the Arab scholar and traveller Al-Masudi, having chanced into Daghestan, wrote delightedly about "meadows of gold and springs of jewels" and said that the country was inhabited by "seventy races and tribes, each with its own customs, language, and king." Indeed, Daghestan remains the most multinational of all Soviet republics. In its territory at present are eighty-one nationalities, speaking seventy languages and dialects.

There is a legend which the Daghestanians tell (and it is told by other Caucasian peoples as well) explaining the incredible variety of languages in their land. God, it is said, was carrying all the languages of the world in his arms to distribute to different peoples. When he was crossing over the Great Caucasian Range, he tripped on Mount Elbrus, spilling all these tongues into Daghestan, on the other side of the mountains.

Caucasian languages have long been a puzzle to linguists. With the exception of Osset and Armenian (Indo-European) and Azerbaijanian (Turko-Tatar), the Caucasian languages are all unrelated to any living European or Asiatic languages. Marr, the controversial Russian linguist of the Stalin era, attempted to link the different Caucasian languages with Basque. However, this line of thinking has long since been abandoned. To make things even more difficult for scholars, the Caucasian languages are etymologically unrelated and mutually unintelligible.

TABLE 2: Languages Spoken in the Caucasus

Indo-European	Iberio-Caucasian	Altaic	Semitic-Hamitic
Slavic	Northwestern group	Turkic	Assyrian
Russian	Abkhasian	Azerbaizhanian	
Ukrainian	Adygian	Karachaev	
Armenian	Cherkessian	Balkar	
Iranian	Kabardinian	Kumyk	
Ossetian	Central group	Nogai	
Kurd	Chechen	Turkmen	
Talyshian	Ingush	Tatar	
Tat	Tushin	Kazakh	
Farsi	Northeastern group	Mongol	
Greek	Avar	Kalmyk	
Greek	Darginian		
	Lezgin		
	Lak		

At the present time, there is a tendency toward the merging of nationalities, at least administratively and economically, although linguistic problems are still great. However, many groups are multilingual. For example, among the small group of Archis, in addition to their native language which they use in everyday life, many speak Russian, Avar, and Lak, the languages of their neighbors. Close trade relations with neighboring groups contributed to the spread of a number of languages.

Schools, the economy, and political organizations have all helped to increase the knowledge and use of the Russian language. Since the Caucasus became part of the Russian Empire, and especially in the Soviet period, Russian is required in the schools and is the administrative and official language. But at home and with friends, Caucasians speak their native tongues. While some of the old people understand Russian but speak it with difficulty, the young people raised under Soviet rule understand it very well.

Peoples which lacked a written language have had alphabets devised for them by Soviet linguists. Since then, newspapers and books in the local languages have enjoyed a tremendous growth. Nations having written languages of their own, such as the Georgians and Armenians, have kept them.

The Northern Caucasus experienced a much greater Asian nomadic influence on language than did Transcaucasia, which had close contact with Iran and Turkey.

Linguists call the native Caucasian languages "Ibero-Caucasian." The intriguing name, Iberia, was introduced by the ancient Greeks who called the Caucasus "Eastern Iberia" and what is now Spain and Portugal "Western Iberia." As far as we know now, the Ibero-Caucasian languages originated and were developed by the aboriginal populations.

The Caucasian languages are distinguished by an abundance of consonants; Cherkess, for example, has fifty-seven. Some words contain long sequences of consonants which are difficult for a European to produce. For example, Abkhasian has five manner series: labialized, palatalized, glottalized, aspirated, and voiced in eight positions of articulation. To an outsider, the speaker of Abkhasian seems to be producing a series of gentle explosions, although the vowels are expanded in singing. The sounds include a wavering trill, whistling noises, and a prolonged buzz. The languages are highly guttural, a Semitic characteristic.

The vocabularies reflect the people's immediate concerns. There are great elaborations of words dealing with pastoralism and with wild and domesticated animals. Since wild plants are an important part of the Caucasian diet, there are many words naming and describing the properties and stages of growth of plants. Kinship terms, especially for patrilineal relatives, abound. This is in keeping with the patrilineal, patrilocal way of life.

The combination of anthropological, linguistic, and historico-ethnographic evidence makes it clear that this is an ancient population of probable common origin with great cultural continuity, vitality, and resiliency. Caucasian peoples have resisted linguistic and cultural assimilation by the many intruders and newcomers in their area.

RESETTLEMENT

Natalia Volkova has studied a specific instance of a process familiar throughout the Caucasus—the resettlement of a primarily cattle-breeding mountain people into the plains regions and their transition to an agricultural economy. Her study involved peoples of the Northern Caucasus—Karachai, Balkarians, Ossetians, Chechens, Daghestinians—inhabiting the area of the Great Caucasus Range from the northwest to the southeast.

According to the economic report of 1882, these mountain regions (excluding Daghestan) were over 657,748 desiatinas (an old land unit) in area, but only 5,445 desiatinas were under cultivation; less than 1 per cent of the territory was useful for agricultural purposes. This inadequate amount of agricultural land could not even supply the mountain people with bread year-round; they were often forced to buy their bread from the plains people. Such a situation was characteristic of the Northern Caucasus during several different historical periods. Every available plot of land was utilized. The size of land-measuring units indicates the small dimensions of these agricultural plots: the *aiak-uzun* and the *tashorun,* Balkarian terms meaning "a foot's length" and "the area under a single stone."

The difficult agricultural situation in the mountains of the Northern Caucasus created the problem of surplus population. According to the Abramovsk Commission (1907–1908), the surplus was 67 per cent among the Balkarians, 88 per cent among the Ossetians, 89 per cent among the Ingush, and 90 per cent among the Chechens. This surplus was forced to work as hired laborers or to resettle in the plains.

Surplus population may also explain the extreme militarism of the Northern Caucasus, a phenomenon which became amply evident to the Russians during the Caucasian War when the Northern Caucasian peoples resisted fiercely. Fighting was an easy and natural occupation for people without work and beset with economic difficulties. Peter the Great, after visiting Daghestan in 1722, said: "If these people had an understanding of military art, not one nation could compete with them."

The Georgians did not develop such aggressive militarism, nor did they glorify thievery as did the small northern groups. While the aggressive, militaristic opposition of the Northern Caucasus was dealt with severely by the Russians, both before and after the Revolution when whole groups from the region were exiled, the Georgians retained their national autonomy.

Militarism in the Northern Caucasian was also abetted by the absence of a class of skilled craftsmen such as existed in the South. The lumpen, un-skilled, and unemployed population was fertile ground for a strong military class and its concomitant machismo philosophy.

The fanatic acceptance of Islam in the Northern Caucasus was a further factor aggravating this militaristic machismo. The poverty of the region was a vital precondition for the spread of Islam, and the religion's proselytizing character provided an ideological justification for militarism, conquest, and plunder.

The lack of arable land in the mountains was the basic reason for the resettlement of the mountain people in the plains where there was still unoccupied land. This process proceeded most energetically from the second half of the eighteenth through the nineteenth century. The many Daghes-tanian settlements in the plains testify to the migration of extended family clans *(tokhums)* from the mountains.

After the annexation of the Caucasian regions in the middle of the nine-teenth century, the Russian government encouraged the resettlement of mountaineers to the plains. The Russians felt that they could then more easily control the rebellious mountain people.

One witness of the resettlement process among the mountain Ossetians in the 1880s wrote: "The resettlement from the mountains to the plains is accomplished quite easily in the following manner. A mountain dweller seeks a wife among families living in the plains and temporarily settles at the house of his wife's relatives. After a year or so of living off the hospitality of his new family, without any prior warning the mountaineer would build a dwelling in some unoccupied place in the village, supposedly for his new wife's family, and then move his whole clan down from the mountains permanently." After some time, this same account tells us, "the newcomers would appear before the village and demand a part of the common lands."

The Soviet authorities took upon themselves the task of redistributing land to the people, a measure which was taken from 1926 to 1928. As early as 1920, temporary measures had been taken to provide local populations with land. Redistribution was indispensable, since at the very beginning of Soviet rule, the landless mountain people had begun to swarm en masse to the plains. Along with the redistribution of privately owned lands came the expropriations of lands from the most affluent villages and regions. Thus, the Karachais received several plains regions of Kabardinia and the Piatigorsk Region of Tersk District. In 1922 to 1923, Daghestan A.S.S.R. received a large part of Kisliarsk District and Achikulaksk Region.

In the autonomous republics of the Northern Caucasus, the redistribution of land was closely tied to the resettlement of mountain people in the plains. This migration led to the formation of a number of new settlements.

Not all of the resettlements of these years were successful. The Daghestanians met many difficulties on the plains, including new climatic conditions. Malaria, however, was the greatest tribulation, causing many to return to the mountains.

Since the Revolution, many new settlements have been made in the autonomous republics of the plains by settlers from the mountains. There are still very few roads in the Northern Caucasus, a problem which has plagued the area since before the Revolution. But urbanization increased the intercourse between city and village, making medical care, manufactured products, and culture available to the indigenous population as well as to the newcomers. In past years, thanks to the construction of a number of irrigation canals, it has been possible for settlers to build larger and better collective farms, to develop economically, and to produce new crops such as grapes, garden vegetables, and rice.

Various ethnodemographic changes—equally important results of resettlement—occurred, particularly the widening of the territories of a number of ethnic groups. The Ossetians, Chechens, and Ingush broadened their territory during the eighteenth and the first half of the nineteenth century. The Karachaians, Laks, and Darginians expanded their territory during the Soviet period. In addition, the ethnic composition of a number of Northern Caucasian regions changed. For example, the Khasaviurtovsk and Caspian plains regions near Kizliar were settled by Avars, Laks, Lezgins, and Darginians. New multinational villages developed in which daily contact between many different peoples made possible the cooperation and rapprochement of cultures and languages, with a concomitant development of linguistic abilities among the population.

HOUSING

In housing there is tremendous variety in style and materials, depending on the ecology and the history of the area. A prime consideration was protection from raids and blood feuds.

For example, until a few decades ago, most Abkhasians built wattled huts which in time of danger could be quickly taken apart and transported in a two-wheeled cart drawn by an ox or a donkey. Home sites were selected for minimum visibility at a considerable distance from each other, because of fear of attacks from neighboring tribes and cattle thieves, and of attempts to take prisoners for sale into slavery.

In some of the isolated highlands of Georgia, stone fortresses of three, four, or five stories were built close to each other, creating a defensive wall. Modern architects marvel at these monumental structures, which must have been designed by expert builders.

Each floor had a special purpose. The ground floor served as a sanctuary for children and women during wars. The men defended them from the upper floor. There was a floor for animals, and a place for provisions to be stored for beasts and people. Grains, dried fruits and vegetables, nuts, and so on could last for months. Deep wells supplied water. There were openings in the walls for shooting; ammunition was stored nearby. Some villages were surrounded by battle towers on all sides, and the towers for habitation were between the battle towers.

Feuding families used to retreat to their fortresses. Usually, each fortress belonged to a specific lineage. Behind the fortresses were houses built in ascending levels. Each house was tightly abutted to the next and the roofs of the lower houses served as terraces for the upper houses. Now the Abkhasian wattled huts and the towers serve mostly as extra storage space, and the fortresses as tourist attractions and points of pride for local patriots.

The towers were constructed largely with boulders taken from mountain springs. Only at the corners does one find hewn blocks—massive ones. The work of master masons is apparent in the careful clay-plaster mortaring between the stones. The larger gaps between the boulders were filled with smaller stones from the river bed. The walls are secured with separate flat flagstones which extend within the towers at an angle. During construction, external scaffolding was not utilized; the towers were constructed from within. The construction of the scaffolding paralleled the tower construction.

The towers do not have foundations, but are placed directly on the cliffs or on slate bedrock. The Vainakhs chose the tower site by pouring milk over the ground. If the milk did not soak into the earth, the site was considered a good one. Construction commenced and the first row of stones was reddened with the blood of a sacrificial sheep. Although earthquakes are not rare in the mountains, the towers, despite their seemingly primitive construction, continue to stand.

Construction was not supposed to take longer than a year. The person for whom the tower was being built was required to feed the workmen well. According to legends, hunger was the root of any misfortune occurring during the construction. For example, if a workman were to fall from the tower because of dizziness, the person for whom the tower was being built would be accused of stinginess and driven from the village.

The craft of tower-building was passed down from father to son. The Ingush Berkinkhoev family from the village of Berkin, still well known as master builders, has constructed towers even outside the borders of Ossetia. In the Khevsursk village of Akhieli stands a tower constructed by the Ingush at the price of fifty cattle.

Formerly, most homes were stone in the mountains, wooden in the forest areas. They were rather simple, often lacking a chimney; smoke escaped through windows and doors. Some people had small caves which formed the center around which the rest of the house was built.

In the Moslem areas, women and children had quarters separate from the men's. In addition, there was a guestroom or *kunac* (meaning "friend") for male visitors. Friends were received in this room. Women could bring food there for the guests but they never took part in the entertainment of visitors. Even people who were not well-to-do tried to have a guestroom, both as a necessity and as a status symbol.

Furnishings were of the simplest kind. Wooden platforms ran along the wall, with pillows thrown against them for comfort. Small tables with short legs were used to serve food. In poorer homes, food was spread on cloths on the floor and people sat cross-legged around the cloth while eating. Only in better homes did people sleep on linen; in poorer homes, rags were thrown on the floor for sleeping.

Even now, Caucasian people do not accumulate possessions. The homes are not crowded with furniture and gadgets, but, with the increased affluence of the collective farms, factory-made furniture is used. The people now have kerosene, coal, and wood-burning stoves. Many now have tables and chairs. One even occasionally sees a television set or a radio. Record players and records of native songs or Russian music are very popular. Still, in some areas (for example in Armenian villages) work is done sitting on the floor. There is little furniture in village homes.

Interior structures have also undergone a change. Instead of a separate outside entrance to each room, there are now interior doors. Rooms previously lacked doors because the women's quarters were always separate from the men's and only the husband or father was permitted to enter the women's quarters.

There are now many similarities with Russian construction. Many prefabricated sections are used. The traditional Caucasian *kunac,* previously for men only, is now being gradually transformed into a living room for both men and women.

Daghestanian dwellings have always been poor because of the poverty and severity of the land, the absence of wood in large areas, the comparative isolation from the outside world, the traditional asceticism of the mountain people, and the constant warfare.

INDUSTRIALIZATION

Urbanization and modernization have transformed many villages. According to the 1970 census, Georgians lead the Caucasian region in urbanization while the Avars in Daghestan are the least urbanized.

In the Caucasus, industrialization brought the greater accessibility of consumer goods and mass culture. Except in certain urbanized areas, such as Baku, industrialization was not the same socially disruptive process that it was in the West or even in other parts of the Soviet Union. Industrialization meant mechanization of farm work, not a sudden exodus from rural areas into the cities and the disruption of traditional society.

THE MOUNTAIN JEWS

Most Jews in the Caucasian Mountains live in Daghestan and Azerbaijan, although separate groups also live in the cities. In the past, they lived mostly in the mountains, and it is from this that they get their name. In the eighteenth and nineteenth centuries, they began to move into the valleys. Now they live in settlements in Madzhalis, Mamrach, Zhanzhal, and Kala and in the cities of Derbent, Machachkala, and Buinaksk (Daghestan), as well as in a number of other cities of Azerbaijan. The largest number of mountain Jews live in the cities of Groznyi and Nalchik. According to the census of 1959, there were 15,000 mountain Jews living in Daghestan and 10,000 in Azerbaijan. The population has since greatly increased.

The mountain Jews are ancient inhabitants of the Caucasus. Their forebears settled in southern (Iranian) Azerbaijan, where they adopted Tat language (a dialect of Iranian) although retaining their Judaism. In this area, they intermingled with the native population. During the fifth and sixth centuries A.D., they settled in the Caspian lowlands. Then began their gradual ascent into the mountains and the formation of a separate culture.

The mountain Jews are an agricultural people. Their early agricultural methods were extremely primitive, combining labor and magic, and were geared to their own use rather than for external sale. They grew wheat, rice, peas, melons, cabbage, onions, and so on. Plowing and planting were done by men, weeding and harvesting by women. At the beginning of the season's work, there was the singing of ritual songs mentioning the different stages of work. Dry areas were irrigated by canals from nearby rivers but the peasants also often used magical rituals to bring rain. It was their custom not to go back for those plants which were left unintentionally after a harvest. Instead, poor people were allowed to collect them. This custom, called *khushe,* also applied to the harvesting of fruit.

Rice was a very important part of the diet of the Jews. There was never a holiday or festivity without rice. Cultivating rice is one of their most ancient occupations. All hard labor connected with the rice paddies was performed by men. Women participated in the preparation of the paddy for planting and then in weeding.

Many Jews also worked in the production of silk and tobacco. Since not everyone owned land, many people worked as laborers for others.

Another very old occupation of the Jews was the cultivation of fruit. In the nineteenth century, grape cultivation was so widespread among Jews that those who had very little land neglected the cultivation of grains and devoted themselves exclusively to grapes. There were approximately twenty varieties of grapes. The Jews also grew tree fruits, especially apples, pears, cherries, and plums.

The mountain Jews are known as very good tanners. They make soft and excellent leather. They also are dyers, tailors, and hat-makers. In addition, there were many craftsmen in what is known as cottage industries, which brought very little income; the craftsmen lived at a bare subsistence level. In the cities, before the Revolution, they were small merchants.

The Jews resembled their neighbors in housing, in farming, in clothing, and in many other ways. But, probably because of the difference in religion, the

Jews segregated themselves in one section of a village or city, where they tried to keep their dietary laws. They did not eat pork, nor did they eat horsemeat, a frequent part of the Azerbaijan diet. In any case, meat was not readily available to poor people. Sugar, also, was used only when a guest came or on holidays when every dish was accompanied by tea.

To this day, the mountain Jews preserve the patriarchal extended family, which is called *tukhum* or *taipe*. These terms are now used for people who have the same family name and remember some distant forefather is common.

Judaism forbids Jews to marry those of other religions. Men were allowed two wives. This practice was found among wealthier people and among some rabbis, especially if the first wife did not produce offspring. The wife had no rights whatsoever, but was completely subject to her husband's wishes—like chattel property. He could divorce her at any time but she could not divorce him nor did she receive an equal inheritance.

Parents usually selected the mate, giving much attention to material conditions. Paid marriage brokers were employed. The groom was supposed to pay a bride price to the bride's family. Children were sometimes betrothed.

After the bride's family consented, the groom's family began preparations for the betrothal ceremony. On the day of the betrothal, the groom gave a number of gifts to his future bride, including a white silk kerchief and a wedding ring, which was ceremoniously brought to her home by the women of his family. The ceremony took place at the bride's home. A procession headed by the oldest members of the groom's family proceeded from his house to the bride's, sometimes accompanied by music. In her house, the closest relatives and friends of the bride were assembled. After the ceremony, there was gaiety, music, and dancing. The old people seated at separate tables were honored by special toasts and speeches.

There was sometimes a period of several years between the betrothal and the wedding. During this period, the young people exchanged gifts and made offerings of various kinds of food and drink. When meeting the relatives of the groom, the bride would hide or cover her face with a kerchief. The young man did the same to avoid meeting the bride's relatives.

The actual wedding usually took place when the girl was fifteen or sixteen and the boy seventeen or eighteen. Relatives on both sides, especially aunts and uncles and brothers and sisters of the young couple, helped make the arrangements. A week before the wedding, the family of the groom notified the bride's family that they were beginning their preparations. Many guests were usually invited, including relatives, friends, musicians, and neighbors.

Celebrations were held simultaneously at the bride's and the groom's homes and lasted for three or four days. (Generally, the whole ritual of marriage has been greatly influenced by Caucasian customs.) When the celebrations near the end, the groom and his family and friends come to fetch the bride. She was dressed in her very best attire and surrounded by her girl friends. Her face was covered with a kerchief. As she was led out of the house, both processions joined together and proceeded with music and torches to the synagogue where a ceremony was conducted under the *khupa,* and then on to the groom's house.

On this last evening of festivities, the groom's parents held a feast to which everyone was invited. After the evening's celebrations ended, the guests went home and the young couple was shown to the nuptial chamber.

Shortly after she went to live with her husband's family the young wife assumed the same work responsibilities as the rest of the family. After her first child was born, she no longer needed to hide her face in front of her husband's older relatives.

There is a marked difference in the treatment of children, depending on their sex. Boys bring greater rejoicing than do girls. Children usually receive names taken from the Bible, but a boy may be given his grandfather's name.

One of the ancient customs of the mountain Jews, as well as of other Caucasians, is hospitality. They have always entertained many non-Jews. Wealthier families had a special guest room where the guest enjoyed finer linen and better food than did the rest of the family.

Most Jews were poor and lived in very small quarters where hygienic conditions were rudimentary and diseases were rampant. Infant mortality was especially high. Like their neighbors, the Jews blamed bad spirits for much disease. The only protection they felt they had were talismans. They shared many pagan beliefs with all other Caucasian mountaineers.

After a death, men and women took part in ritual crying. The deceased was buried without a coffin on family land. In the house of the deceased, prayers were said for the departed soul and food was distributed. For forty days, the closest relatives were in deep mourning. Even the poorest family tried to put at least a small monument on the grave.

In pre-Revolutionary times, most mountain Jews were illiterate. There were some synagogue schools and private tutoring from rabbis. Only boys could study and their knowledge was limited to the memorization of religious books. Disobedient boys were beaten. There was no secular education and only a few boys from wealthy families went to schools in Baku or Derbent.

The Socialist Revolution brought great changes.

Jews began to work in new and different areas. They became technicians and industrial and skilled workers. A considerable portion of their working force is now made up of women.

In general, the Jews have better living conditions now. They have two-story houses with windows. They have radios. Many places have electricity. But some peasant families still sit on the floor and eat from a cloth even though there may be a table and chairs in the room. The old custom of sitting on pillows or mattresses and eating at low tables also remains.

Food is prepared according to the Caucasian Jewish tradition. Despite the fact that the collective farms bake bread, the Jewish members prefer to bake their traditional bread in special ovens, called *ton*. A favorite dish is made of lamb, rice, and vegetables, and they still make chopped fish in the European style. However, the Azerbaijan cooking has influenced them; the dishes are very spicy. There are two dietary innovations: special food for children, and the increased use of sugar and other sweets.

Forced marriages no longer occur. Young people often choose their own mates. Polygamy has been abolished. Sororate and levirate marriages are rare. Large extended families no longer live together because of migrations to the cities and employment away from the family land.

Cultural differences between the villages and the cities have also been reduced. Formal education and the appreciation of the arts, such as theater, are increasing.

There are many very old individuals reported to be among the Mountain Jews. So far very little research has been done on them and the ages of the longevous people were not verified.

3

ARE THEY REALLY THAT OLD? THE DEMOGRAPHY OF LONGEVITY

THE CONCEPT OF OLD AGE

The average American family moves, we are told by statisticians, once every five years—a very short time for a family to put down roots, preserve its past, or develop meaningful, continuous relationships with others in the community. An older person moving into a new community is at the greatest disadvantage, often meeting with the indifference of people who lead more active lives and who have no reference to his past.

Growing old in the community where one was young creates a continuum made up of many small and large ties, so that the old person is much more than his aging self—he is the sum total of his life. His past exists in the memory of the community, which sees him as what he is and as what he was. And so does he. Children of his contemporaries, and their children, and even their children's children can relate to him in ways that strangers in a new community cannot. He can expect visits from youngsters who will listen to his stories of the past because it is *their* past as well, who will eat his cookies, or ask for a Band-Aid or comfort.

This brings to mind the small island off the coast of Maine where I spend summers when I am not on another continent. There are many elderly people on the island who were born and grew up there. I spent some time with one of them, a 101-year-old man, Arthur Spurling (called Chammy), who lived in a spacious two-story home which he maintained himself, keeping it in immaculate condition. I visited him for tea and he served cookies which he himself had baked. The year before, when he became a centenarian, the whole village had celebrated his birthday at a party, which pleased him very much. On his hundred and second birthday, another party was given to which most of the village came. A friend in the village called me in New York the next day. "Poor Chammy," she said. "After the guests left, he was getting ready for bed, took off his trousers, collapsed, and died."

A neighbor of mine in the same village, a woman of almost ninety-three, Saidi Fernald, was often visited by children and youngsters who enjoyed her stories of the past. She crocheted and did handwork for people in the village. Although she enjoyed television, she much preferred the company of people who dropped by.

Longevity is not uncommon on the island. On the contrary, examination of the town clerk's records and the stones in the cemetery shows a high percentage of natives who live well into their eighties and late nineties.

A rural village anywhere, of course, has certain elements in common with the regions of the Caucasus we have been describing—a slower pace, a regular rhythm in the activities of life, a certain interdependence of neighbors and family, and a continuity of relationships from birth to old age. The pressures and fragmentation of urban life simply preclude a functional, harmonious place for old people. But, like the Maine island, there remain rural corners even in our own country where the old are valued and able to maintain their dignity and usefulness. In such places, there seems to be a higher proportion of long-lived people who are healthy and productive.

What are the upper limits of human life? There is a raging controversy on this subject among the scientists. Some believe that there is no proof that any human ever lived past 113. Others claim to have known of people 160 years and more. It has been estimated that during the Paleolithic period the average life-span was 26 years. In the Neolithic the life-span increased to 32 years. During the early historic period—fifth through ninth centuries A.D.—it reached 36. In 1900 the average Russian could expect to live 48 years and the average American 47 years, but by 1975 the average life expectancy at birth had increased in both countries to 74 years.

I always find it curious to encounter, as I often do, skepticism as to the authenticity of the ages of the long-living people of the Caucasus. Indeed, it often seems to me that the doubters actually do not *want* to believe that people live to such great ages anywhere in the world, especially in the Soviet Union. One can, of course, expect to encounter a certain degree of disbelief among those who have never had experience with such old people, but in the face of conclusive documentary evidence, it is hard to explain this stubborn resistance. Could it be that there is a more subtle resistance than that motivated by a healthy scientific skepticism? Are there certain emotionally-charged assumptions which are threatened by the existence of societies where many people live to great old ages in health and productivity? I think so.

The obvious element of envy can be assumed. Everyone wants to live longer. Why don't we, with all our technological and medical expertise? But the issue is much more complex than that.

It would be superfluous to restate here the now widespread indictment of modern, industrialized society and its deleterious effect on the human organism and on its environment. Nor is it necessary to recapitulate the effects of *psyche* on *soma* and vice versa. The simple fact is that all the achievements of Western medical science and technology have not yet been able to show us how to add years of good health and productivity to human life. Indeed, all the discussions of how to improve the "quality" of what we do have inevitably lead us to the uneasy idea that most mechanical efforts to improve people's lives seem to produce the opposite effect. That is, technological inventions to make work easier, potent drugs to cure dreaded diseases, more efficient vehicles to transport us, all seem to have side effects which either complicate our lives further or replace the problem they solve with an even worse one. Typical examples are the anti-cancer drug that may attack and arrest cancer cells but eventually becomes noxious to healthy cells as well, and the wondrous automobile and jet plane that now poison the air we breathe and consume the planet's dwindling fuel resources. The examples are legion and interacting, and we need not catalogue them here. What needs to be said is that there is a growing consciousness that the continued development of technology and modern urban society has brought us to a point of diminishing returns and now threatens our very lives on the planet (and, in fact, the life of the planet itself)—a situation which is indeed disturbing and unacceptable.

In Western societies, old age is essentially a time of retirement from work, physical decline, and social disengagement. In fact, our general dissatisfaction with life may lead to premature aging. This need not be so.

A study of a people who are not only extraordinarily long-lived but who also live gracefully, with dignity, simplicity, and order prompts us to reexamine the treatment of old people in our own society and question some of our basic assumptions about progress. I hope that the description of the lives of these mountain people will have some positive effect on attitudes toward aging and the aged. But I am not trying to prescribe a way of life or to advocate a romantic "back to nature" movement.

Dismissing the evidence of longevity in the Caucasus as Soviet propaganda not only ignores the real evidence but also may be motivated by an anti-Soviet position.

There is even suspicion that Caucasians exaggerated their age in the past for the purpose of escaping service in the Tzarist army. But most of the Moslem tribes of the Caucasus, including Abkhasians, were *not* inducted into the Tzar's armies, being considered disloyal to Russia. Only volunteers were accepted and those, obviously, did not have to falsify their age records. It is interesting to note that the very groups *not* subject to induction into the army contain the highest number of longevous people. There are altogether too many attitudes which militate against a satisfying old age in our society; we should not reject a wealth of material that could show us a better way. That we view longevity as a problem, not the blessing it is among the Caucasians, is in itself a great loss to us.

The cavalier statements of actuarians or statisticians that no man or woman with a verifiable birth record is known to have lived longer than 113 years are insidiously destructive. They set psychological limits, reinforce hopelessness among the old, and contribute nothing to our understanding.

METHODS OF AGE VERIFICATION

It seems to be mere quibbling to discredit reports of longevity by questions about precise ages. If a person lives to 120 rather than 130 in health and vigor, the fact of old age is barely diminished. More telling than even birth records are unmistakable historical connections, the landmarks with which we all punctuate our lives. A Caucasian who fought in the Crimean War would have to be a certain age, within five years or so, to have been in the army at all. (My American assistant, a bit touchy about approaching middle age, laments the fact that her admission that Franklin Roosevelt was first elected when she was a child absolutely precludes her concealing her true age.)

Another point requiring mention about the people in the Caucasus is that they have specific terms or expressions for great-grandparents going back to six generations. These expressions are used to refer to the living, not to those who have died. Very few languages contain expressions for so many generations of living relatives. In Abkhasia, the name for "my great-great-great-grandfather" is *sabdu iab iabdu iab*—six generations. The letter *s* in *sabdu* signifies the speaker. The term for "the son of my great-grandson" is *spa ipa ipa ina*—five generations. *Ipa* means son.

A series of tests of centenarians in 1972 in the U.S.S.R. showed that the people of the Caucasus had the appearance, physical and mental health, vigor, and ability of people about sixty years old. People age at different rates. The mountain people experience their life changes many years later than does the typical Western person. The aging process does not occur uniformly among all peoples. Just as rapid aging may be attributed, in part, to malnutrition or to some other aspect of life-style, slow aging owes something to life-style as well as to genetic make-up.

The medical profession in the Soviet Union has traditionally been very conservative in publicizing cases of unusual longevity. Reports of extreme longevity in the Caucasus were made well before the Revolution, but only in the 1930s, with the interest of the gerontologist A. A. Bogomolets, did Soviet medicine begin systematic studies of longevity. One of the areas which had earlier been reported as having many long-living people was Yakutia, in Siberia. Gerontologists and anthropologists were dispatched on an expedition to investigate these reports and concluded that they were unfounded. Conservatism generally has been the rule in the evaluation of cases of extreme longevity by the Soviet medical profession.

The Gerontological Center in Georgia, under the direction of Professor G.Z. Pitskhelauri, with the cooperation of local health centers and medical doctors, made detailed medical examinations of the long-living. Altogether 15,000 people aged eighty and over were examined. In accordance with the study design prepared by the Institute of Gerontology and Experimental Pathology of the Academy of Medical Sciences in the Soviet Union, great attention was given to logistic verification (mobility) and the correlation of reported age with birth certificates, passports, and records of the collective farms. The ages of the long-living were also correlated with those of their children, grandchildren, and great-grandchildren. The data were analyzed with the help of a control questionnaire.

The ages established for the calendar year 1968 were correct in 2,681 instances, or 66 per cent. An error of from three to ten years was found in 836 instances, or 31.1 per cent, and errors of more than ten years were found in seventy-seven cases, or 2.9 per cent. For 120 long-living people, the age established was much higher than the one reported in the census. In the Georgian census of 1959, there were 2,080 people (790 men and 1,290 women) aged one hundred and over. That means fifty-one people per 100,000.

It should be noted that cases of extreme longevity in the Caucasus have been observed by the most prominent Russian gerontologists. In 1904, the father of modern Russian gerontology, I.I. Mechnikov, met a Georgian woman reported to be 180 years old in the city of Gori. In 1937, A.A. Bogomolets, founder of the world's first institute of gerontology, personally investigated twelve Abkhasians from ninety to 142 years of age and found no pathological organic changes. M. Sultanov, a professor of gerontology and medicine in Baku, personally interviewed and examined thirteen persons from 131 to 167 years of age in Azerbaijan: nine persons 131 to 140 years of age, three persons 141 to 167 years, and one 167-year-old man, Shirali Muslimov, who was until his death in 1973 the oldest person in the world. Professor Sultanov kindly gave me photographs of the people he had interviewed and generously let me read his notes on their lives.

In the All-Union census of 1970 the Bureau of Statistics took measures to confirm the birth dates of all persons over eighty years of age. Since this is a complicated process, the Institute of Gerontology in Kiev expects some inaccuracies in the data and is continuing to make additional surveys. Each person over ninety was interviewed by a local physician; a 272-page manual of specific instructions had been developed for these interviews by the institute in Kiev.

When I first discussed this problem with Dr. Nina Sachuk of the demographic department of the institute, she agreed with me that it is more difficult to establish the correct age of single elderly individuals living in urban centers than of those in rural areas. There the elderly, as a rule, live in the villages where they were born and where they have numerous relatives whose ages are recorded. The verifiable ages of relatives, especially offspring, can be used as a reference point for approximate birth dates (with a slight margin for error) of longevous individuals for whom birth records do not exist.

In Kiev in 1963, a regional European bureau of the World Health Organization established the terminology used today. They decided that the term "late maturity" signifies the sixty to seventy-four age group, "old" refers to persons seventy-five to eighty-nine, and persons ninety and older comprise the "longevous" category.

Doctor of Medicine Ramazan Alikishiev, a noted gerontologist, who did his doctoral thesis on the long-living people in Daghestan, took great pains to establish and clarify the exact dates of birth of the people he studied. He asked the following questions: How old were you during the cholera epidemic in the summer of 1892? . . . at the end of the war of Daghestan against Russia in 1859? . . . the abolition of serfdom in 1869? . . . the mass resettlement of Moslems to Turkey in 1864? He questioned 213 long-living people, seventy-nine men and 134 women in Daghestan. Older relatives of those questioned were of great help in substantiating answers and giving additional details. The gravestones in the local cemetery gave the dates of birth and death. In addition, some parents had written the birthdates of their children on pages of the Koran in Arabic. One man showed Dr. Alikishiev the date of his birth inscribed in thick ink on the ceiling. Most of the people investigated lived in villages with populations of from 150 to 200—village populations never seemed to exceed 2,000. These people generally lived in the same villages all their lives.

It was a small, stable population in which these old people spent their lives. All of them knew the ages of everyone in the village and could easily recite who was older or younger and by how many years. Since respect must be paid by a speaker to his elder, those younger, even by a few years, must be aware of the difference in age. From childhood on, one must learn to show respect even to a brother who is two or three years older. In Daghestan, as in other areas of the Caucasus, all people over ninety form the village Soviet of Elders, which takes part in decision-making for the entire community.

The age of Yanukian Minas Arutiunovich of the village of Mazharka in the Gul'ripsh region was established by this field method. The investigators were told that he was 114 years old. Although he had no birth certificate, there was a record of his marriage in 1863. After a year of marriage, his daughter Varvara (who was still living at the time of the study) was born. She lived in Tsebel'da in the same region. In 1895 his son Akop, sixty at the time of the study, was born. He lived in the same village and had documents attesting to his birth. The old man had ten children, of whom four were still alive at the time of the study, and whose ages were confirmed. He had 104 descendents—children, grandchildren, great-, and great-great-grandchildren. Thus it was confirmed that Yanukian Minas Arutiunovich actually was 114 years old.

The field method of validating age, although painstaking, still appears to be the most reliable. The preparation of family trees, genealogies, and biographical sketches of the aged was very time-consuming but necessary for my study. I could verify the ages of quite a few of the people by visiting the collectives and checking the registers where ages are recorded. In addition, the ages of a number of the long-living people were looked up in the archives where baptismal or marriage ages were checked by my associate, Dr. Grigori Smyr. On the basis of this research, a certificate was drawn up and signed by him and the director of the Institute of Language, Literature and Ethnography in Sukhumi.

One of the people whose age we verified was Vanasha Temur. We visited his home on one of our field trips. He was born in 1867 and lives with his family in the village of Lykhny. As usual we did not announce our visit in advance. As soon as our car stopped at the gate, everyone in the house, including the little children, came out to greet us. Chairs were carried out to the lawn, and we were asked to sit down and be their guests. That meant that we would be entertained and a meal would be prepared for us. Before committing ourselves to being their guests, we asked for Vanasha, their grandfather. They were terribly sorry. Since he had not expected visitors, he had gone to a village about a hundred kilometers away to take part in the wedding of a distant relative. He would be staying there for the two or three days that the wedding lasted. How did he get there? Well, by bus, of course. But maybe we would like to join the wedding guests? They were sure we would be welcome there. I asked what a man 107 years old would do at a wedding. The same as everybody else, they said. He would eat and drink and make speeches and, if he felt like it, he would dance a little!

Temur had a baptismal certificate showing him to be 103. However, he claimed he was christened when he was four years old. Not infrequently, baptism was delayed, sometimes because there was no money to pay the priest. But, as Temur said, there was no hurry. He was not going anyplace. Indeed, he stayed in the same place for all of his 107 years.

We verified that Mkyg Gitzba was born in 1858 in the village of Bzyb, Abkhasia. She was 116 years old when I visited her in October 1974. I saw her in the company of her two daughters-in-law and her son. She was a somber-looking woman of medium height with a full head of gray hair. The weather was pleasant and we sat outside. I noticed that a brick house was being built close by and the second floor had been started. The daughters-in-law were hovering over Mkyg to see that she looked presentable for our pictures, and she was advising them and her son about something in Abkhasian. All I understood was that she was giving orders for a meal to be prepared for us. We immediately declined.

This lady of 116, I was told, sweeps the courtyard (which is of considerable size) every day and looks after the chickens, geese, and other creatures in the courtyard. The impression I got was of someone who is very much in command of what goes on in the household. We did not spend much time with her because we were expected somewhere else and it was getting late.

I intended to return the next day but, as it happened, I did not make my second visit until the end of February 1975. Poor Mkyg was in bed and feeling quite miserable. It seems that one day she wanted to see how much work had been done on the new house and she climbed a builder's ladder—a vertical piece of wood with short horizontal pieces nailed to it. The ladder slipped and she went down with it. Her leg was broken. She was in bed in a very clean room where a wood stove burned and the two daughters-in-law were in attendance. After a few minutes of conversation, Mkyg apologized for being in bed and asked us to stay longer because some food would be prepared for us. She asked us not to photograph her because she looked too miserable. She was sure that the next time I visited, she would be recovered and I could take her picture then.

Another woman whose age we established was Agsha Bartzitz, born May 2, 1870, in the village of Blaburkhua. On my visit in October 1974, she was in excellent health, working hard at keeping house, sweeping the courtyard, feeding the chickens, and so on. (It seems that all the old women worked in the courtyards and certainly the courtyards in Abkhasia were the best-kept I have seen anywhere.) She did not want to take off her kerchief until I offered to comb her lovely gray hair so that she would look presentable for the picture. She looked like a woman of eighty rather than her age. She was a Moslem and was baptized for her wedding when she was thirty-five. There was a baptisimal document to certify it. Her husband was a Christian. They had four daughters and two sons. The youngest son, Kuna, was born in 1907 when Agsha was forty-seven.

A few months later I visited the family again. Agsha was ill with a stroke. She was lying in a tidy bed covered with clean linen and cared for by her daughter-in-law and other female relatives. I don't think she recognized me. Agsha had a younger sister who died a few years ago at the age of 110.

The next day we met Makhaz Lagvilov in the village of Kutol. He was born in 1867 (which made him 108) and christened in the village of Dzherda. He had a baptismal certificate. He married when he was thirty-seven and his wife, twenty-three. They had a church wedding. Eight children were born to them. The youngest son was born when the father was sixty-three and the mother, forty-nine. The son, now forty-five, and his family lives with his father, who is registered at the collective as the head of their household. I asked the old man about his health. "I never showed my body to the doctors, but lately I had to go to the hospital for a few days because of some stomach trouble. I used to smoke heavily. I had a tobacco business, but now I smoke just a little. I did drink, but was never drunk. My eyesight used to be excellent; I was a sharpshooter, could get a bird in flight, and even now I can see very well. But my hearing is not as good. No, I am not married; my wife died some years ago. But you know, all men are the same. I would not mind marrying again. Look at Bzhenia; when his wife died he was 111. He remarried and had two sons. You see, it is very seldom that men get old."

It was verified in 1963 that Kurt Zantariya of the village of Tamish was 119 years old and in very good health. He has an excellent memory for both recent and distant events, remembers the Russo-Turkish War of 1870 (when he was sixteen years old) and relates stories of the Turkish army attacking his region. He remembers well the period between 1864 and 1878, when the Abkhasians were exiled to Turkey. Nine years ago, he became ill and remembers who took care of him and whom he met in the hospital. He recalls that three years ago a Frenchman came through their village and was interested in his life. The man was Gilbert Locke, who wrote about Zantariya in an article called "In the Valley of the Centenarians," which was published in *France–Soviet Union*, No. 152, 1958.

In 1961 Professor P. White also visited this village and proposed in a toast that he and Zantariya be milk-brothers. Zantariya received the toast with great enthusiasm and proposed that their respective countries should be milk-brothers and that there should be no wars between them.

Zantariya worked for many years in the collectives and was given a medal for his achievements. He still works on his family plot, is very clean, and drinks quite a bit of wine at banquets—as many as four glasses. He used to drink more, but says that he was never drunk.

In Georgia, the medical doctors P. Stepanov, C. Stepanov, and M.M. Eiderman of the Social Hygiene Laboratory of Gerontology verified the ages of 2,681 long-living people. Ages were verified by birth certificates, passports, and registers of the village collectives and correlated with the ages of children, grandchildren, great-grandchildren, and great-great-grandchildren and with historical events.

The following account comes from the historian P.G. Butkov. In 1722, during the reign of Peter the Great, the Russians bombarded the Caucasian city of Derbent. The city eventually surrendered. A group of elders went out to meet the Russian authorities. At the head of the delegation was an elder of the City Council who carried a plate on which rested the keys to the city. The man's name was recorded by the Russians. Seventy-four years later, in 1796, a Russian division under the command of General Zubov again stormed Derbent. The city was again bombarded and again it surrendered. A delegation went out to offer the surrender. At the head of the delegation walked an old man, supported by others on both sides. He carried a plate holding a silver key to the city. When the Russians asked him his name, the old man answered that they had recorded it seventy-four years before when he had offered the keys of the city to the officers of Peter the Great. The man was 120 years old on this second occasion.

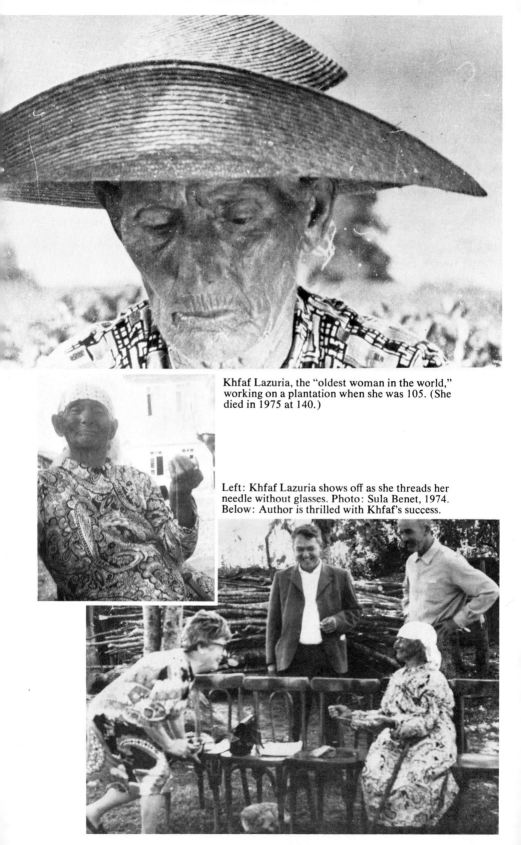

Khfaf Lazuria, the "oldest woman in the world," working on a plantation when she was 105. (She died in 1975 at 140.)

Left: Khfaf Lazuria shows off as she threads her needle without glasses. Photo: Sula Benet, 1974. Below: Author is thrilled with Khfaf's success.

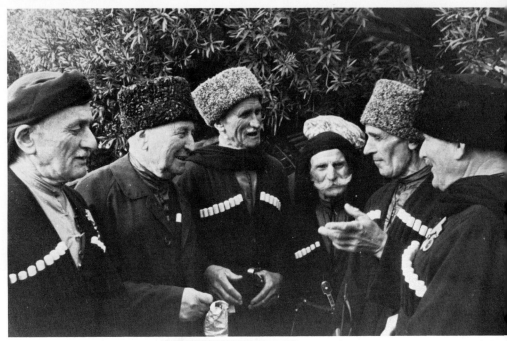

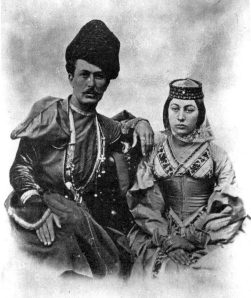

Above: A group of
Abkhasian men
gossiping, 1971. No
one in the group
is permitted
to be under 90.

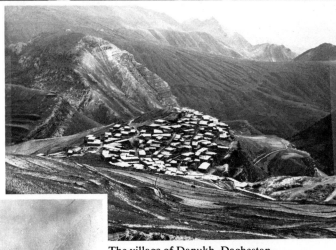

The village of Danukh, Daghestan.

Old Georgian nobility
of the nineteenth century.

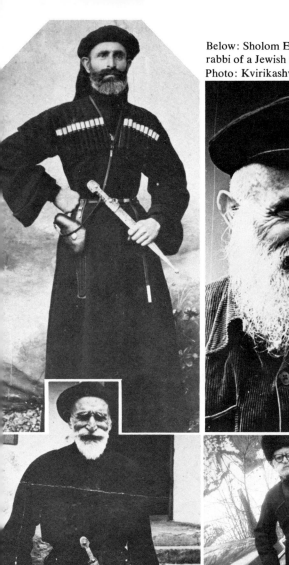

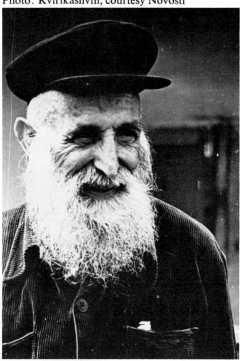

Below: Sholom Eliashvilli,
rabbi of a Jewish village named Tsieteli-gori.
Photo: Kvirikashvili, courtesy Novosti

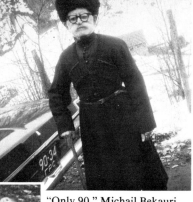

"Only 90," Michail Bekauri
of Pasanauri in Georgia. His father
lived to be 121.
Photo: Sula Benet, 1975

Top left: Shaliman Arshba at 80.

Bottom left: Shaliman Arshba at 127,
shortly before his
death in 1954. He worked as a
mountain guide in
Abkhasia until the
day he died.

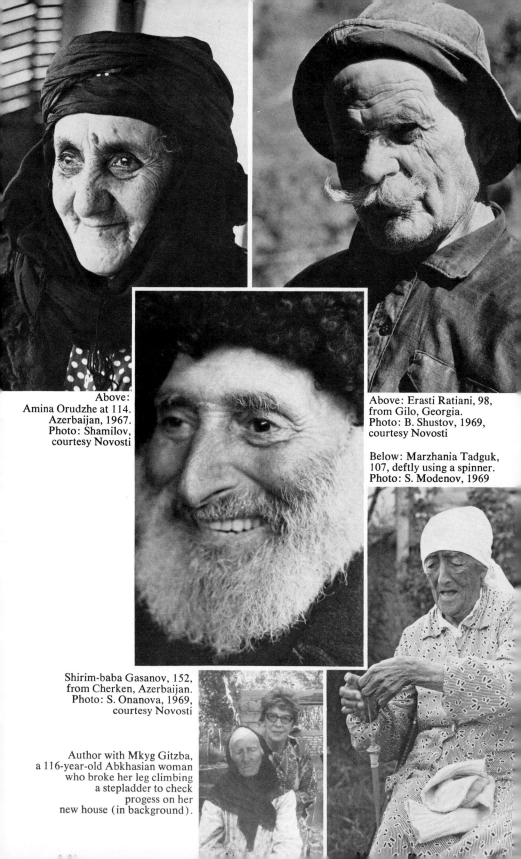

Above:
Amina Orudzhe at 114.
Azerbaijan, 1967.
Photo: Shamilov,
courtesy Novosti

Above: Erasti Ratiani, 98,
from Gilo, Georgia.
Photo: B. Shustov, 1969,
courtesy Novosti

Below: Marzhania Tadguk,
107, deftly using a spinner.
Photo: S. Modenov, 1969

Shirim-baba Gasanov, 152,
from Cherken, Azerbaijan.
Photo: S. Onanova, 1969,
courtesy Novosti

Author with Mkyg Gitzba,
a 116-year-old Abkhasian woman
who broke her leg climbing
a stepladder to check
progess on her
new house (in background).

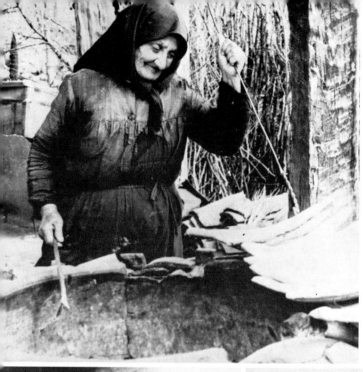

Mauke Ekvshaureshvili,
born in 1860,
from Nakartzeli, Georgia.
She is baking bread:
the long, thin loaves,
slightly curved
at the ends, are
characteristic of
eastern Georgia.

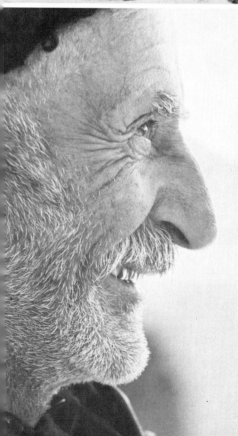

Gidaat Sarkerov, over 100 years old, from
Khynalyg, Azerbaijan. Photo: Abramochkin,
courtesy Novosti

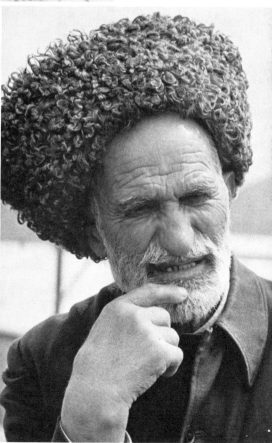

Gusein Kurtul, 96, from Daghestan.
Photo: I. Ozerski, courtesy Novoski

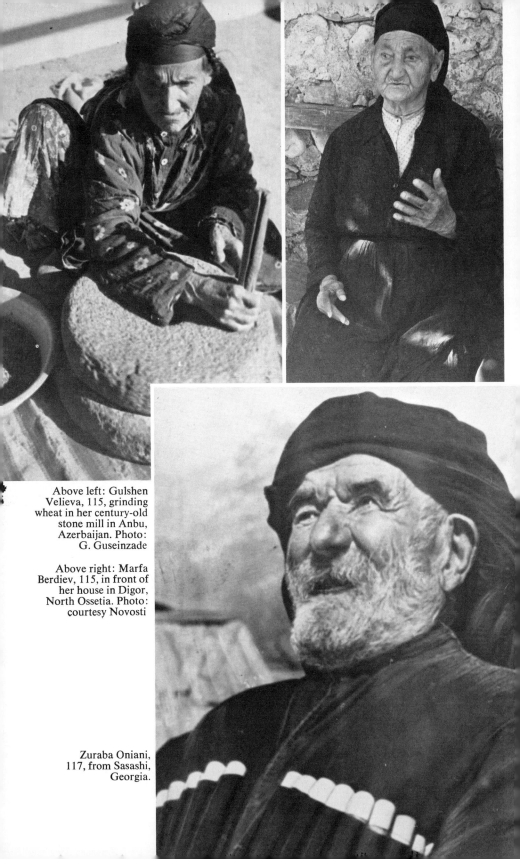

Above left: Gulshen Velieva, 115, grinding wheat in her century-old stone mill in Anbu, Azerbaijan. Photo: G. Guseinzade

Above right: Marfa Berdiev, 115, in front of her house in Digor, North Ossetia. Photo: courtesy Novosti

Zuraba Oniani, 117, from Sasashi, Georgia.

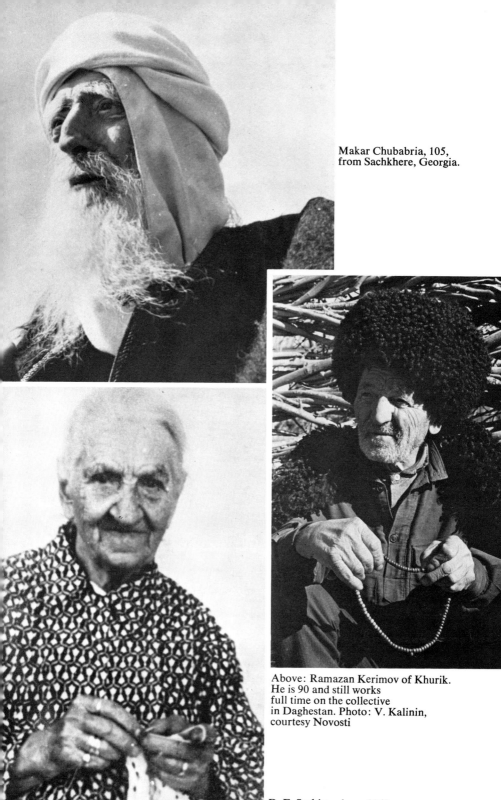

Makar Chubabria, 105,
from Sachkhere, Georgia.

Above: Ramazan Kerimov of Khurik.
He is 90 and still works
full time on the collective
in Daghestan. Photo: V. Kalinin,
courtesy Novosti

D. F. Sarkisev, born 1861,
in Batum, Georgia.

Right: Aligishiev Goitemir at 97 in 1972. He is wearing a winter coat called a "guala." Tsilitl, Daghestan.

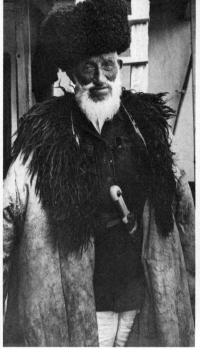

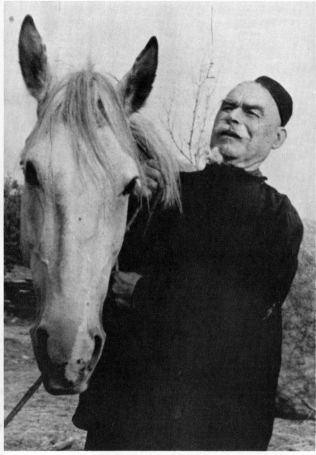

Left: Dzhauakhishvili, born in 1866. Digomi, Georgia.

Below: Kruashvili and Moisashvili, both born in 1862. Georgia.

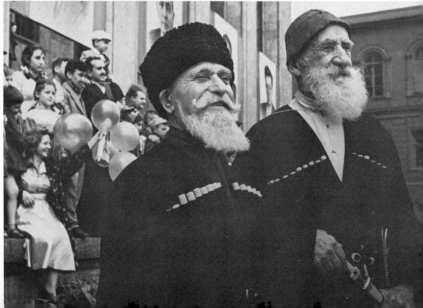

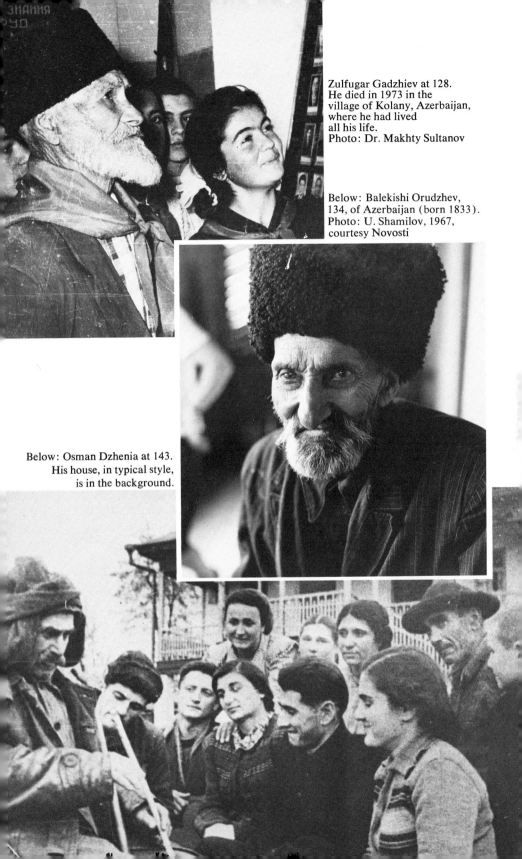

Zulfugar Gadzhiev at 128.
He died in 1973 in the
village of Kolany, Azerbaijan,
where he had lived
all his life.
Photo: Dr. Makhty Sultanov

Below: Balekishi Orudzhev,
134, of Azerbaijan (born 1833).
Photo: U. Shamilov, 1967,
courtesy Novosti

Below: Osman Dzhenia at 143.
His house, in typical style,
is in the background.

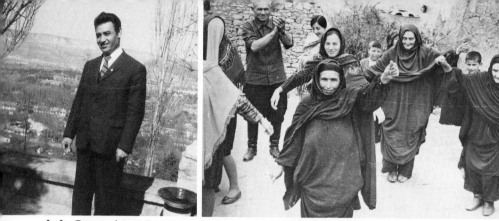

Left: Gacan, the modern groom, at his wedding. Photo: Sula Benet. Right: Dancing at a traditional wedding. Old women lead the dance in which all ages participate. Daghestan, 1972. Photo: courtesy Academy of Sciences, Moscow

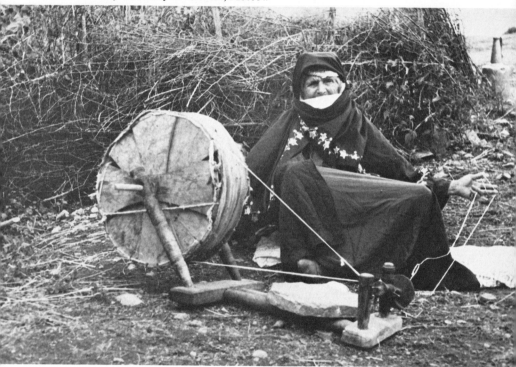

Above: A. T. Gregoran, an 86-year-old Armenian woman, spinning. (The mouth covering is removed only to eat, and then inconspicuously.)

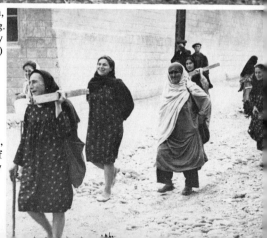

Women going to work in the field. Gergebim, Daghestan. Photo: courtesy Academy of Sciences, Moscow

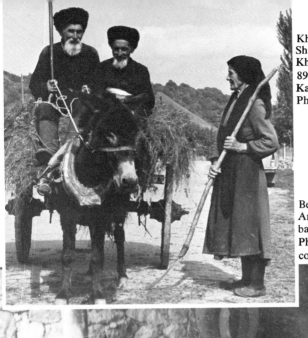

Khasan Tumenov, 106, on the left;
Shakhbaz Kurukov, 118, on the right;
Khasan's wife, Napifkhai,
89, standing. Babugent,
Kabardino-Balkaria, Northern Caucasus.
Photo: Dr. M. Sultanov

Below:
Armenian woman and daughter-in-law
baking bread. Porbi, Armenia.
Photo: A. Ter-Sarkisiants,
courtesy Academy of Sciences, Moscow

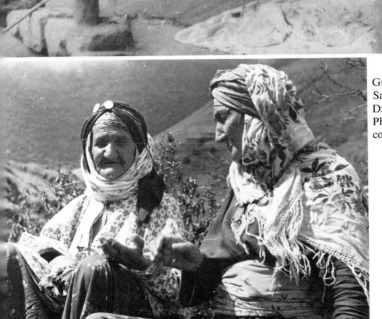

Gulbaidshi Gusein, 112, left;
Sanam Aliev, 102, right.
Dzhoni, Azerbaijan.
Photo: Kalinin, 1974,
courtesy Novosti

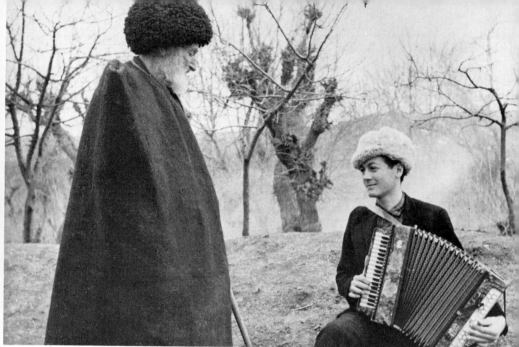

Above: Shirim-baba Gasanov, 152, listens with pleasure to contemporary music. Azerbaijan, 1969. Photo: courtesy Novosti

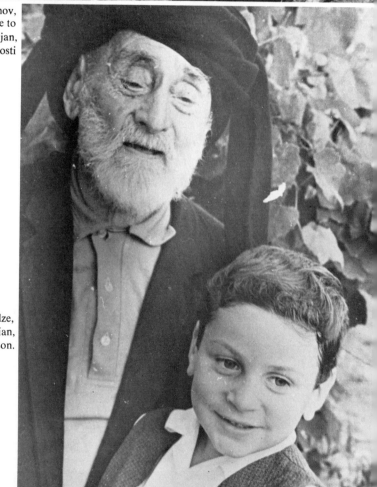

Suleiman Bezhanidze, 100-year-old Georgian, with his grandson.

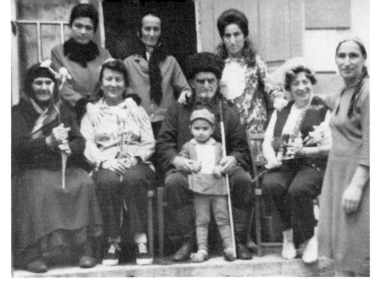

Semenlary Bekirbi, 108, center; his wife, far left, is 98; the woman on the far right and the one standing at center are his daughters; the two other standing young women are his granddaughters; on the old man's left is Dr. Vera Rubin, Director, Research Institute for the Study of Man, New York; on his right, the author. Zolikokoazhe, Balkaria, North Caucasus, 1973.

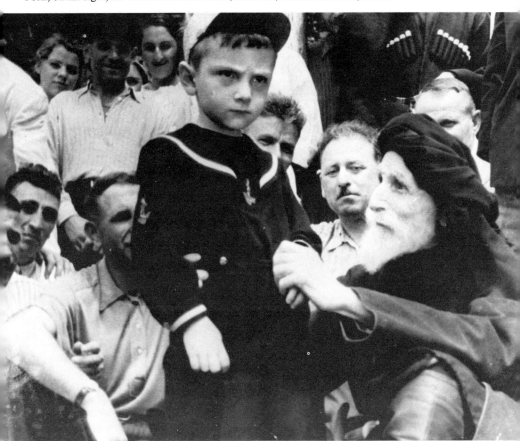

Suleiman Arshba, 122, at right. Trvarcheli, Georgia.

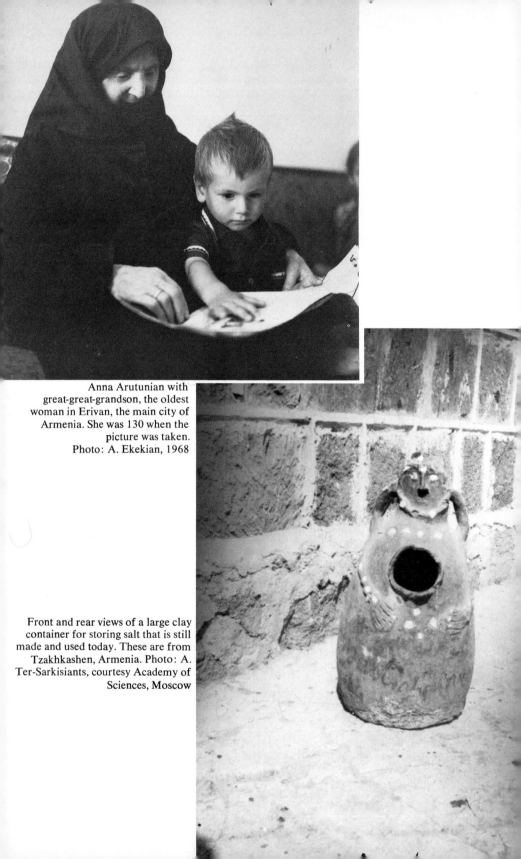

Anna Arutunian with great-great-grandson, the oldest woman in Erivan, the main city of Armenia. She was 130 when the picture was taken. Photo: A. Ekekian, 1968

Front and rear views of a large clay container for storing salt that is still made and used today. These are from Tzakhkashen, Armenia. Photo: A. Ter-Sarkisiants, courtesy Academy of Sciences, Moscow

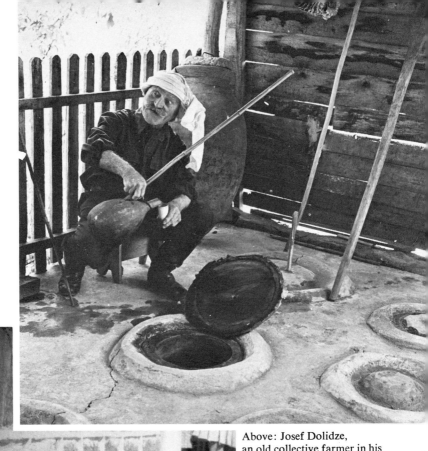

Above: Josef Dolidze,
an old collective farmer in his
marani (wine cellar).
Every respectable
villager should have a *marani*.

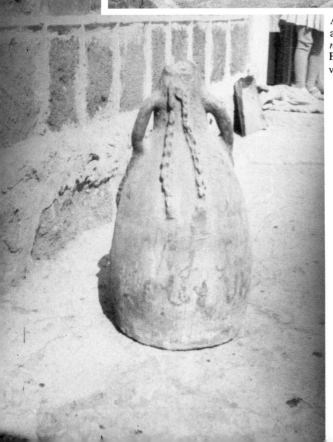

Tskhenburti, the Abkhasian horseback game.

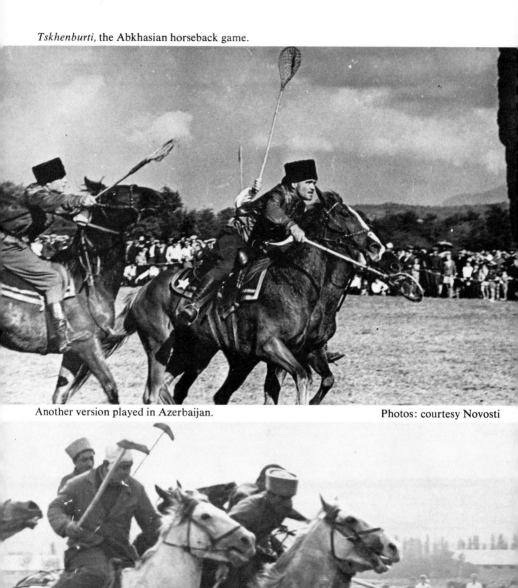

Another version played in Azerbaijan.

ECOLOGICAL ZONES

Demographic studies based on the All-Union census of 1959 and 1970 indicate that the distribution of the longevous population in the Caucasus is far from uniform among the republics and even within a single republic. There are also striking rural-urban differences and differences between mountain, foothill, and plains regions. Almost all long-living people are permanent residents of rural areas. In the cities, the longevous population is made up of either isolated cases or newcomers from villages.

According to an analysis made by R. Alikishiev, based on the 1959 census, there are four times as many long-living persons in the mountains of Daghestan (1000–4500 feet above sea level) as there are in the valleys or plains. The difference is striking. In the Gumbetov region of the mountains, for every 10,000 individuals, there are seventy men and 117 women who live to ninety or older. In the Kazbek region in the foothills adjacent to Gumbetov, this proportion drops to fifty-three men and 106 women. The lowest index of longevity is found in the plains, where for every 10,000 individuals, only 4.8 men and twelve women live beyond ninety.

In B.G. Kindarov's study of differences in health and mode of life among long-lived individuals of the Checheno-Ingush Republic in the Northern Caucasus, three ecological zones were distinguished: the mountains, foothills, and plains. The study included approximately 470 individuals of ninety and older, and about 4,000 members of their families. There were dramatic differences between individuals of different ecological zones and between men and women, in physical activity, interest in life, and mental disposition.

Kindarov found that both men and women in the mountain regions are

TABLE 3: Health (percentage rated "good") of people ninety and older, in various zones of the Chechen-Ingush Republic

Sex	Zone	Activity	Capacity for Self-Aid	Interest In Life	Good Mood
Male	Mountains	83.3	83.3	58.3	45.4
	Foothills	72.2	77.8	44.4	41.2
	Plains	41.6	61.5	16.7	33.3
Female	Mountains	56.1	71.9	12.9	34.5
	Foothills	46.2	44.8	13.8	26.9
	Plains	33.3	54.5	9.0	20.0

far more active, have more capacity for self-aid, are more interested in life, and are more likely to be in a "good mood" than their counterparts in the plains regions. Foothills men and women were on a slightly lower level than those of the mountain regions. "Good mood" means positive mental disposition; "self-aid" means elementary functions such as dressing oneself, washing, eating, mobility, and so on. Kindarov believes that a partial explanation of these differences can be found in the life-styles in the zones. The overwhelming majority of long-lived men in the mountain zone (83 per cent) were employed in pastoral and agricultural work during their youth, maturity, and even old age. Animal herding demands both strenuous physical activity (a great deal of climbing and walking) and an unhurried pace of life.

The incidence of diseases associated with advancing age varies greatly from region to region and in different ecologial zones. For the year 1964, the Bureau of Statistics gave the following figures for Daghestan:

TABLE 4: Incidence of Diseases, Daghestan, 1964 (per 100 thousand persons)

	Mountains	Foothills	Plains
Strokes	4.1	7.3	46.8
Heart attacks	0.17	0.2	1.2
Hypertension	13.0	38.8	80.6

There were ten times as many strokes (due to arteriosclerosis of the brain) in the plains as in the mountains, and seven times as many as in the foothills. There were six times as many heart attacks in the plains as in either the mountains or the foothills. There was six times as much hypertension in the plains as in the mountains, and twice as much as in the foothills.

One can see a marked correlation between Kindarov's findings and the figures of the Bureau of Statistics. The plains people, having the least activity, capacity for self-aid, interest in life, and least positive mental disposition, have the highest incidence of strokes, heart attacks, and hypertension.

Medzhid Agaev, age 133, is an Azerbaijan shepherd for the village of Dikaband. He is still working for the collective. He drinks only spring water and yogurt diluted with water. Four times a day he eats small portions of goat cheese, honey, vegetables, and fruit. He does not smoke or drink wine. Following his herds he walks no less than ten to twelve miles daily with his sheep.

SEX DIFFERENCES IN LONGEVITY

In the Caucasus, as in most of the world, more women live to old age than men. But signs of aging—such as wrinkles, poor posture, loss of hair, and difficulty in movement—are more evident in women than in men. Men move with lighter step, are more erect and keep their narrow waists much better than women. Old men like to wear their traditional Caucasian coats fitted snugly at the waist and drawn tight with a narrow belt. Old men's coats are usually quite worn out and have been in the family for generations. Apparently the men's figures remain almost the same as when they were young. This cannot be said of most women, although both men and women are rather thin. In Georgia, I did see some very old people who were obese, but these were exceptions.

In an interesting study on the question of relative longevity in men and women, Dr. N.N. Sachuk, using data published by the U.N. and covering the period 1900 to 1965, examined life tables of most of the countries of the world. She found that in the countries with longer life-spans, the differential between men and women is greater than in areas showing shorter life-spans. That is, in countries where people live longer, a greater percentage of women survive men than in those countries where life-spans are generally shorter.

The data of a special medico-social investigation of 40,000 persons aged eighty or over, carried out in various geographical and economic regions of the Soviet Union, shows that the health of longevous women as compared with that of men is not as good. Old men have better mobility, self-sufficiency, and their eyesight and hearing are better preserved. Longevous men report fewer diseases in their medical histories than do women.

To explain this seeming paradox, Sachuk suggests that since there are higher mortality rates among men aged twenty-five to thirty-four and fifty-five to sixty-four, only the healthiest survive to advanced age. In women of these earlier age groups, the mortality rate is lower, so a relatively larger number of women survive to longevity. But, as the data also shows, it is men who reach *maximum* longevity, not women.

No hard scientific conclusions can be drawn from any of Sachuk's data, but from the studies of the Caucasus which presently exist, the following may be said:

1. In the Caucasus (as in the rest of the world), a greater number of women than men survive to old age.

2. In the group of longevous Caucasian people, *up to the age of a hundred,* the men, though fewer in number, possess better health and physical capacity.
3. Men attain *maximum* longevity in greater numbers than women; that is, after the age of a hundred, an *increase* in the relative number of men is observed.

These facts suggest that the process of natural selection operates strongly in the question of male longevity, and less so in female. This would explain the greater health and strength of longevous men in relation to women, and the men's attainment of maximum longevity in greater numbers than women. The genetic and environmental factors which kill more men than women at an earlier age insure that only the "strongest" men survive to old age. Sachuk also mentions that longevous men in the Soviet Union have long-living relatives, a fact pointing to genetic heritage as significant in longevity.

THE GENETICS OF LONGEVITY: IS AGING GENETICALLY PROGRAMMED?

Only some longevous people have relatives eighty or over. Abkhasia has considerably more longevous people than the Ukraine, but fewer of them are related to each other. Is longevity in Abkhasia determined by genetic factors or by something else? In Daghestan only 47.5 per cent of longevous persons had close relatives who also lived more than a hundred years.

Both women as a group and the Caucasus as an area have lower correlations than the Ukraine between longevity and close longevous relatives. More comparative study is necessary, but this may indicate that in the Caucasus, longevity results from the *absence of deleterious influences,* while in other areas longevity appears to be tied to genetic factors.

In the study of materials from Azerbaijan S.S.R. and Kabardinian-Balkar A.S.S.R., we often come across families and clans of long-living people. Thus

TABLE 5: Long-living Relatives (80+) for each 100 persons in the "old" and "longevous" age groups, by sex

Territory	Men		Women	
	80–89	90+	80–89	90+
Ukrainian S.S.R.	61	66	57	62
Abkhasian S.S.R.	57	61	46	53

Nurdzhakhan Pirumovaia of the village of Aidynbulag, Vartashenskii Region, Azerbaijan S.S.R., has five longevous sons, 109, 107, 105, 98, and 92 years. But it should also be remembered that in families of six to eight or even ten to twelve children, often only one, two, or three are long-living.

The significance of the genetic factor in longevity remains unclear.

In discussing the effect of genetic factors on longevity in the Caucasus, it must be remembered that in a society where the children adhere to the life-style of their parents, emulating them in all practical things such as diet, exercise, and so on, it may very well not be a question of genetic inheritance at all. It may simply be a question of culture and environment.

In considering the genetics of longevity in the Caucasus, one must look at the rules of marriage which operate in each group. In Daghestan and Azerbaijan, marriage was traditionally contracted with close relatives, namely cousins (both parallel and cross cousins). By contrast, the religious laws of Georgia and Armenia did not permit marriage to kinsmen. The Armenian National Council of 365 A.D. prohibited all marriages in the lateral line up to the third degree of relationship. Other church decrees and traditions considered marriages between relatives even up through the seventh degree incestuous. Marriage between people who have the same family name is considered by Abkhasians to be incestuous. Formerly such a marriage was punished by the expulsion of the couple from the village or even by death. The social prohibition against these marriages is still just as strong, although, of course, the punishment has been abolished since criminal law is now administered by the Soviet courts. It is important to note that in Abkhasia, an area with one of the highest longevity rates in the Soviet Union, marriage is always contracted outside the family. Thus, hereditary causes cannot be credited here. As far as is known, there is no specific gene for longevity.

DEMOGRAPHY OF LONGEVITY AND HEALTH STANDARDS

Several republics famed for unusually high longevity were selected for study: Azerbaijan S.S.R. (including Nakhichevan A.S.S.R. and Nagorny-Karabakh A.R., Georgian S.S.R. (including Abkhasian A.S.S.R., Adjarian A.S.S.R., and South Ossetian A.R.), Armenian S.S.R., Daghestan A.S.S.R., and North Ossetian A.S.S.R. They afford an extraordinary opportunity for correlating cultural patterns with longevity, since they are of different historical backgrounds, religious beliefs, and physical types. Georgia has been Christian and literate since the fifth century, the Daghestanians and Azerbaijanians are zealous Moslems of the Shiite order, and the Abkhasians less ardent Moslems of the Sunni order. The last three groups began to write their native languages only under the Soviets.

Villages with high percentages of long-living people are clustered close together so it is possible to study a number of villages, their inhabitants, and the historical-genealogical connections within a relatively brief time.

At what age do the Caucasians consider themselves or others to be "old"? I asked people of different age groups and, in the replies, I found that the idea of chronological age was seldom mentioned. As long as a person is active, functioning, and capable of participating in the life of the family and community, he is not old, whatever his years. People think of themselves as being old only when they no longer are able, physically and mentally, to take part in the activities to which they have been accustomed.

In rural areas, there is an extremely wide range of activities: one moves from the strenuous labor of youth into the less physically demanding tasks of very advanced age.

The vigorous appearance of old people in the Caucasus makes it extremely difficult for Western observers to estimate their age. From their appearance, it is hard to say whether they are seventy or twice that age; close to 40 per cent of aged men (over ninety) and 30 per cent of aged women are reported to have good vision; that is, they do not need glasses for any sort of work. Between 40 and 50 per cent have reasonably good hearing. Most have their own teeth. Their posture is unusually erect, even into advanced age.

One man of 107 said "I am not old yet. I am in good health and working. I will be all right yet for a long time to come." In the Caucasus, people feel that as long as they are in good health, working, and functioning in their social roles, they are not old. Nevertheless, they insist on receiving honors because of their chronological age and their important place in the family and the community. Whenever an old person was spoken of to me, he or she was referred to as "The Honorable so and so. I soon recognized that "honorable" stands for old age.

On the collective farms men over sixty and women over fifty-five receive small pensions. They usually continue to work full time although with age their work diminishes. Almost all of the old people I interviewed, even those far over one hundred, continued their work in the collective. Since they are paid by the days that they work and since they are not afraid of being fired, there is no competition for their jobs. They work at their own pace.

LONGEVITY AND FAMILY LIFE

Significant numbers of individuals over one hundred are found only in those areas of the Caucasus where the extended family still exists and still functions, and where the long-living are heads of or important members of such families. There is a positive correlation between large families and longevity. Such has been my observation in Abkhasia and in parts of Azerbaijan, Karachai, and Chechen-Ingush. I have been told that it is also true in Daghestan. In areas of comparatively short life-span—the Baltic republics of Lithuania, Latvia, and Estonia; some regions of European U.S.S.R., the Ukraine, Byelorussia, and R.S.F.S.R.—families are significantly smaller. The following table compares family size among the Caucasian, European, and Ukrainian republics of the U.S.S.R. for the year 1959.

TABLE 6: Family Size, per 1,000 Families, 1959

Republic	2 to 3 persons	7 persons or more	Average size of family
Ukrainian S.S.R.	554	33	3.5
Lithuanian S.S.R.	558	43	3.6
Latvian S.S.R.	671	18	3.2
Estonian S.S.R.	695	14	3.1
Georgian S.S.R.	455	84	4.0
Azerbaijan S.S.R.	379	161	4.5
Armenian S.S.R.	309	194	4.8

The high respect accorded to the long-living in the Caucasus is not accompanied by ancestor worship, nor is there suspicion that the old people may be involved in witchcraft. When old people appear in folklore, they are usually benevolent figures.

An elder person was always invited to grace the table at all the dinners I attended. If an elder was not in household, someone was sent to find an elderly distant relative to fill the role. I was impressed by the tremendous stamina of the elderly and by their ability to outdrink me on all occasions.

Loneliness—the Russian term *odinokij* means living alone—among the aged is considered a special problem by gerontologists. It leads to a general dissatisfaction with life and not infrequently to what is considered premature old age—before the age of seventy-five. As a rule, old people living alone are subject to greater economic hardships than are those living with their families. They also exhibit higher rates of digestive disorders, coronary arterio-sclerosis, hypertension, and diseases of the central nervous system.

In the U.S., John Collette, a University of Utah sociologist, found that loneliness was more dysfunctional to health than was overcrowding, and that people who live alone are far more vulnerable to hypertension, ulcers, neuroses, excessive drinking, and drug use.

Loneliness in the U.S.S.R. is more frequent in the cities than in the villages and reflects the tendency toward urban generational family division.

TABLE 7: Frequency of Loneliness Among the Elderly

Republics	Per 100 persons aged 60+	
	Town	Village
Russian S.F.S.R.	11.18	10.67
Ukrainian S.S.R.	10.80	9.90
Byelorussian S.S.R.	10.37	10.28
Modavian S.S.R.	10.03	14.03
Lithuanian S.S.R.	15.95	20.37
Latvian S.S.R.	25.00	19.96
Estonian S.S.R.	27.21	28.25
Georgian S.S.R.	8.65	8.59
Azerbaijan S.S.R.	9.07	.7.20
Armenian S.S.R.	4.83	7.56
Uzbek S.S.R.	7.12	4.94
Kirghiz S.S.R.	6.21	4.86
Tajik S.S.R.	6.07	4.18
Turkmen S.S.R.	7.64	5.26
Kazakh S.S.R.	5.62	4.76

A recent study conducted by Y.K. Sokolov of the Medical Institute in Chelyabinsk, U.S.S.R., found that big-city living damages the health of elderly and aged persons. In larger cities, cases of hypertensive diseases and diseases of the nervous system are more frequent. People living on streets with heavy traffic are more likely to complain of headaches, sleeplessness, heart pain, and indigestion than are those who live on lanes or quiet streets.

THE GROWTH AND REPRODUCTION CYCLE

The over-all length of life is determined by the length of the individual periods or phases of life—infancy, childhood, youth, maturity, aging, and old age. In each period, the possibilities and reserves of the following periods are determined.

Children develop much faster now than forty or fifty years ago. The difference begins in the weight of newborn babies, which has increased 100 to 300 grams. The birth weight doubles in four months—an increase that used to take six months. Teeth erupt one to two months earlier. Pre-school children are ten to twelve centimeters taller than in the last century. Sexual maturity is earlier.

In the past century, growth continued until age twenty-six. In 1940, it continued until age twenty-one. Today, boys between eighteen and nineteen, and girls between sixteen and seventeen stop growing.

The reasons for this acceleration are not known. Possibly a better diet is an contributing factor. The consumption of meat (especially pork), fat, and sugar has increased. A meat diet stimulates endocrine function, which is important in growth. Climate, physical constitution, and the growth of technology also play major roles.

Low metabolism can be correlated with low maturation, and could naturally prolong the entire life process. Animals with low metabolism are known to have a long life expectancy.

The connection between late menarche, late menopause, and longevity deserves attention in future research. I have seen only one report of such research in Soviet literature. However, my impressions were reinforced by my discussions with workers in the medical profession.

I also had an opportunity to interview a group of rural high school girls in the Republic of Balkaria, a region known for longevity. Most of the girls reported menarche between the ages of fifteen and sixteen or later—a few at seventeen. In contrast, in the city of Tbilisi, Georgia, as reported by Dr. B.C.

TABLE 8: Age of Women at the Birth of Their Last Child and the Presence of Longevous Relatives in the Family Genealogy

Group Under Study	No.	Age at the birth of the last child		X^2
		under 42	over 42	
Those not having longevous relatives	540	525 (97.2%)	15 (2.8%)	$X^2=5.6$
Those having longevous relatives	220	203 (92.3%)	17 (7.17%)	P 0.05
Those having longevous mother	130	124 (95.4%)	6 (4.6%)	$X^2=4.4$
Those having longevous father	53	45 (84.9%)	8 (15.1%)	P 0.05

Solov'eva, menstruation began between twelve and fourteen years of age, but there was no substantial difference between Russian and Georgian girls in the city.

Late menopause is also observed in areas of marked longevity. Ramazan Alikishiev, an internist and noted gerontologist working in Daghestan, reported that between 1969 and 1972, 1,000 children were born to women over fifty and even as old as sixty. Physicians in Abkhasia told me that it is not uncommon for women of fifty to fifty-five to give birth.

Examples of prolonged fertility were given me by good friends who are members of the Amichba family of Sukhumi. The two sisters and two brothers helped me with my work. They are university-educated people, very much aware of the necessity of supplying accurate figures. The sisters, attractive unmarried women in their early forties, with no lack of acceptable suitors, were postponing marriage until their eldest brother chose a wife. Abkhasian tradition dictates that older brothers and sisters marry first. The Amichba sisters felt that postponement of marriage until later in life would pose no problems as far as child-bearing was concerned. They had the example of their two maternal aunts who married late, even for Abkhasians. Their Aunt Dzhgug, at fifty, married Tamshuk Ashula, seventy; it was the first marriage for both. They had two sons, and both parents are living and in good health. The second aunt, Dzab, was married two years later, also at age fifty, to Petra Kapba, seventy. They had a son and a daughter. Both children are now in their late twenties and their parents also are alive and doing well. "From mature parents come well-formed children" is the Abkhasian saying.

Interesting clinical observations on the relation between longevity and the reproductive function were made by L.F. Kovalenko of the Institute of Gerontology in Kiev. According to his data, women now in the 80 to 104 age group had borne twice as many children as had women in the sixty to seventy-nine age group—an example of the unusual fertility of the longevous women. Kovalenko studied women who bore their last child at the age of forty-two or over. The longest child-bearing period was noted among women having longevous fathers. Those having longevous mothers had only a third as many children. Women whose longevous relatives were more distant had half as many children as those who had longevous fathers. Women with no longevous relatives at all had only a fifth as many children at forty-two and older.

B.G. Kindarov reports that in Checheno-Ingushetia the long-living come from families in which the average age at marriage, the number of children, and the age of the parents at the birth of their last child are characteristically high.

Of long-living men who have many offspring, I can mention the following: Magomed Nurmagomedo, (130) of the village of Lower Mulebki in Sergokalimki region with eighteen children, twenty-one grandchildren, and eight great-grandchildren; Mekhmud Alieo (106) of the village of Gunei in the Tabasaranski region with six children, twelve grandchildren, and fifteen great-grandchildren. Among the women are Ashura Murtazaeva (106) in the village Urkarakh in Dakhadaevski region, with thirteen children, twenty grandchildren, and ten great-grandchildren; Aurinat Omarova (120) of the village Mazhab in Charodinski region, with ten children, twenty grandchildren, and twenty-nine great-grandchildren; Khadizhat Magomedova (105) of the village of Kozeda in the Kakhibski region, with eleven children, twenty-six grandchildren, and twenty great-grandchildren; Ashrat Besenaev (110) of the village of Dylym in Kazbek region, with eight children, thirty-three grandchildren, and thirteen great-grandchildren; Balakhany Aslanova (120) of the village of Zue in Tabasar region with fourteen children, sixty grandchildren, and 180 great- and great-great-grandchildren; Shavzade Shikhanova (101) of the village of Gurisa in Tabasar region, with ten children, thirteen grandchildren, and fifteen great-grandchildren.

The unusual fertility of Gadzi Murtazaliev, a man who married for the third time at the age of ninety and subsequently fathered thirteen children, was explained by his wife, Zagidat, as due to his good humor. He never cursed, even when exasperated. He considered a peaceful life, without quarrels, the greatest blessing.

The last children were born for men between the ages of 93 and 104 in a few cases, and for women as old as 60.

Professor Dzidzeria, head of the Institute of Literature in Sukhumi, once agreed to lend me his car for a trip to a distant village. He said that the car was very weak but told us that if we made it up to the village of Tamysh we should visit Georgi Bzhania, the headmaster of the village school. Georgi's father, Ashkhangeri, had lived to be 146. Professor Dzidzeria had known him well and had been invited by the old man to be present at Georgi's wedding. As is usual at Abkhasian weddings, hundreds of people were present. Professor Dzidzeria said: "Since I was Georgi's professor, I was treated with great respect, and the older Bzhania often came to talk with me in the course of the evening. At one point, I said to him: 'They say you have lived through four emperors. Which do you think was the best?' The answer was immediate: 'Alexander the First.' 'Why?' 'Because I was young then.' "

I arrived at the home of Georgi Bzhania with two friends. We were greeted by Georgi, his wife (who teaches in the village school), and his daughter (a student at the Pedagogical Institute in Sukhumi). They were delighted to have unexpected guests. Although we had said that we could stay for only a short time and that we had eaten before we came, dishes of nuts, a compote of damson plums, wine, home-made fresh goat cheese, bread, and whatever else they had in the house were brought to the table. Finally we could not resist and tasted some of the food.

I took a great liking to the family. The wife was charming. She was not as slim as Abkhasian women generally are. I have noticed that the younger generation is much plumper than the older. Georgi Bzhania was a striking man, resembling the actor Yul Brynner. I asked him if he had a good recollection of Ashkhangeri and he said he did. At Georgi's birth, his father was 110 and his mother was forty-six. He recalled that his father was usually in excellent health and quite elegant looking. I had also heard from other people that Ashkhangeri was always well-groomed. He washed himself with cold water every morning and dressed carefully. People said that he always looked much, much younger than his age.

Ashkhangeri Bzhania was married twice. His first wife bore him seven daughters and one son. His second wife had two sons; the older is fifty and the younger, Georgi, is forty-eight. The father had a herd of sixty or more sheep. Every summer he pastured them in the mountains, which he climbed with great ease. He had tremendous physical strength and was also known as an excellent horseman and marksman and hunted a great deal. During the collectivization period he became a member of a collective and was employed in growing corn. He slept outside on the open porch all year round. He was a Christian and took part in the Russo-Turkish War of 1877. When the Abkhasians were given the option of emigrating to Turkey, he refused.

We had to cut short our conversation because it was getting dark and we had a two-hour drive to reach the city. Our hostess brought out packages of tea, nuts, flowers, and their heavenly tasting tangerines, all of which we loaded into the car. Just before we drove away, Georgi invited me to stay with them for three months, since they had an extra room upstairs. I said that I couldn't promise to stay for three months but that I would be delighted to stay for three days if they would have me.

Certain dates in Ashkhangeri Bzhania's life have been verified by the Gerontological Institute of the Ukrainian Academy of Sciences. In 1937, some members of the academy visited him and recorded their conversation. Ashkhangeri told them that he remembered very well the construction of the Georgian Military Road in 1842. He said that at the age of sixty when he married a woman of thirty, "my beard was already gray." He lived with his wife for fifty years. Of their nine children, four were still alive in 1956.

Of good character and respected by the villagers, he liked to socialize, was popular, did not quarrel with people, and did not like being alone. He ate everything, including meat, but in the summer he preferred vegetables and milk products; during the winter he ate more meat. He very seldom ate or drank anything hot. He drank wine in moderation, and was never drunk. From the time he was very young he smoked, but stopped at about the age of 128. His hearing was not very good by then and he also complained about his memory. "Imagine," he said, "I put something down and then I don't remember where I left it!" He had considered himself old only for the past six years because his lower legs, below the knees, had become weak. He still had all his teeth. He died in 1947 at the age of 146.

Dr. Vera Rubin had come to the Caucasus to visit me and to observe, if possible, the longevous people at first hand. On a lovely summer morning at five o'clock, the *babushka* who looked after us woke us up to say that a car was waiting. The trip was a surprise. It was arranged on a day's notice by Vladmir of the Intourist in Kislovodsk, in the Northern Caucasus. He had heard Dr. Rubin express a desire to interview centenarians. But we were not told of our destination. We thought we were simply going to tour the area. Instead we were taken to the mountain village of Zolykokoazhe, in Balkaria, to meet one of the long-living and his family. There we met Semenlary Bekirbii, 109 years old. He read his holy Koran every day without glasses and slept on an open porch in both summer and winter. His great-granddaughter, the village teacher, told us that until five years before he still hunted. She described with great admiration how he could shoot straight, never failed to bring down his quarry, and hunted during most of his life. He was a blacksmith by occupation until he was 104 years old, when his work impaired his hearing; otherwise, he considered himself to be in good health. He was extremely attentive during our visit and very conscious of his own person and dignity.

We had entered the profusely carpeted, well-furnished cottage wearing shoes, which we carefully scraped before entering. However, when we noticed that all the women in the house were in their stocking feet, we apologized and offered to remove our shoes. But one of the daughters said, "Please don't worry. We are going to scrub up after you leave."

The old man's wife, Khytai, was an energetic ninety-six-year-old woman with jet black hair, very lively black eyes, wearing several layers of garments. She seemed to be very much in charge of the whole situation. As we asked questions, Semenlary Bekirbii occasionally looked toward her. She was all smiles and obviously enjoyed all the attention. However, when Dr. Rubin asked who made the decisions in the family, the great-granddaughter immediately answered: "*Dadu* (great-grandfather) of course!"

Dr. Rubin, noticing that he had a watch at his waist, asked Bekirbii for the time. In a very slow and deliberate motion, he pulled out his time-piece, considered it carefully, and answered correctly without putting on eye-glasses.

INDEX OF MAXIMUM LONGEVITY (IML)

Dr. N.N. Sachuk of the Institute of Gerontology in Kiev and her staff analyzed data from the All-Union census of 1970 and developed the Index of Maximum Longevity (IML). This is a tool for the statistical evaluation of high levels of longevity in a given population. Sachuk hoped that in addition to discovering the natural human age limits, the IML would reveal a whole spectrum of factors affecting longevity as well as permit recognition of local patterns of longevity. The IML is the number of persons 110 and older divided by the number of those 100 and older, multiplied by 100:

$$\text{IML} = \frac{\text{number of individuals 110 and over}}{\text{number of individuals 100 and over}} \times 100$$

Only areas containing several hundred persons a hundred and older are suitable for this analysis. Each longevous population was divided into four sub-groups—urban men and women and rural men and women—which had previously been demonstrated to manifest substantial differences in longevity.

The IML ranges from 0 in Estonia to 19.8 in Northern Ossetia (that is, there are almost twenty persons of both sexes of 110 years and older for every 100 people of one hundred years and older). Azerbaijan, Georgia, and Armenia have IMLs of over 10. Abkhasia, Nakhichevan, Daghestan, Kabardino-Balkaria, and Chechen-Ingush show high indices in the range of 12 to 20.

Despite the fact that there are more longevous women than men in the under-one-hundred age group, the 1970 census shows more men than women over one hundred. For the U.S.S.R. as a whole, the IML for hundred-year-old men is 11.4 $\pm$ 0.5, which is almost a third more than the IML for hundred-year-old women (8.1 $\pm$ 0.2).

LONGEVITY QUOTIENT

Soviet scientists have calculated the ratio between the number of people over sixty and those ninety or more. This is the longevity quotient or LQ,

TABLE 9: Geographic Distribution of Long-living People in the U.S.S.R. (Ratio of those 90 + to those 60 + [x/100], based on the All-Union Census of 1959)

Regions	Ratio
I. Transcaucasia	
Nagorny-Karabakh A.S.S.R.	59.6
South Ossetian A.S.S.R.	50.9
Nakhichevan A.S.S.R.	48.1
Abkhasian A.S.S.R.	40.1
Adzharian A.S.S.R.	32.7
Armenian S.S.R.	24.8
II. North Caucasia	
Daghestan A.S.S.R.	39.2
North Ossetian A.S.S.R.	33.2
Kabardino-Balkaria A.S.S.R.	31.6
Checheno-Ingush A.S.S.R.	22.5
III. Siberia	
Yakutian A.S.S.R.	33.6
Altai District	19.0
Tyumen District	16.6
Krasnodarsk District	16.5
Kemerovsk District	15.3
IV. Central Asia and Kazakhstan	
Gorny-Badakhshan A.S.S.R.	31.5
East Kazakhstan District	17.6
Tyan-Shansk District	15.1
North Kazakhstan District	15.0
V. European S.S.R.	
Lithuanian S.S.R.	15.7
Gomel District	15.3

expressed as a percentage. For example, in Daghestan, out of every one hundred people over sixty years, 39.2 are over ninety. The LQ is thus 39.2.

LQ can be interpreted as an index of the general health of older people in a particular region or as a projection of life expectancy (having reached sixty, a Daghestanian may consider his chance of reaching ninety as 39.2 per cent).

4

HOW TO BE A PROPER HOST AND GUEST: HOSPITALITY AND ETIQUETTE

Traveler, if you pass my home without stopping, Hail and thunder strike you, hail and thunder. Guest, if my home does not receive you gladly, Hail and thunder strike me, hail and thunder.

The much-admired modern Daghestanian poet Gamzatov found this verse on the door of a house in his village. It reflects the profound importance of the tradition of hospitality throughout the Caucasus. To open one's home to guests and share generously of one's food, wine, song, and even one's possessions is more than just a social obligation; it is the law of the land, a central focus in the life of the community, and a major source of emotional satisfaction and enjoyment.

All Caucasians love their land, and each national group has a legend of its own origin. The Georgian story is that when God was parceling out land to different nations, the Georgians were so busy feasting with their guests that they arrived very late. God shook his head and told them he was very sorry but he had already distributed everything, and there was nothing left for them. "But," God said, "let me think it over. I don't want to leave you empty-handed." The Georgians suggested that God join them at the feasting table with the other guests while he thought it over. God had a marvelous time and was so delighted with the feasting and warm hospitality that he decided to give the Georgians a portion of the land he had reserved for himself! That, of course, was nothing less than a part of the Garden of Eden.

It is sometimes said that the people of the Caucasus live to entertain their guests. There is obviously quite a bit of truth in this. The essence of their culture is manifested in the complex structure of their hospitality. Coming to the feasting table means a great deal more than simply eating; it means partaking of the very heart and life of the community.

The food at a feast is always the very best that can be provided, but the phrasing of an invitation is always "Come and be our guest," never "Come for dinner." The emphasis is on human sharing, not on food. Feasts are occasions for peace-making with enemies, establishing friendships, and creating good-will. Past differences are often resolved, new relationships are formed, and discordant elements are brought into harmony with the well-ordered structure of living so important to the Caucasian people.

It would not be too much to say that the feasting table serves as a training ground for the young. There they receive their richest education in the traditions of their society. They learn to speak eloquently and warmly of their friends and family. The proper rules of etiquette are learned and practiced, later to spread from the table to the rest of life. In most places, young people do not sit at the table when guests are present. They stand around the table in readiness to serve the needs of the adults and to observe the rituals and manners of the feast.

To receive a guest with all possible graciousness, holding nothing back, is a strict moral obligation. Neglecting to do so is a "sin," which brings shame not only to the host himself but also to his entire family and the village. A man could have many virtues, but if he turned away a guest, the whole community would be horrified. On the other hand, a person who is extremely hospitable is known beyond his own village and enjoys great respect. The names of outstanding hosts, past and present, are celebrated in heroic songs.

To this day, a guest in Ossetia is met at the door with words indicative of deep respect for the newcomer and the joy which is felt upon his arrival: "A guest carries a divine blessing." In Abkhasia, a guest is said to bring seven blessings, taking one when he departs and leaving six with the host. Abkhasian men embrace and kiss in greeting. The host makes a circular motion above his guest's head and says, "Let all the evil spirits who may be hovering around you come to me instead." Women greet female visitors by slightly pressing their shoulder against the visitor's chest. Guests not offered these ceremonial greetings may turn around and leave immediately. I myself have never seen a guest leave because of not being offered the proper ceremonial greeting. I was told it can happen, but no one could recall such an incident.

Since each guest is considered godsent, the best of everything is put on the table with the prescribed ritual and ceremony. Even in the poorest family, one gets an elegant reception, although it may involve great expenditures. Relatives and neighbors—indeed the entire community—are expected to participate. According to tradition, it is the neighbor's obligation to contribute food, work, and money, if necessary, for the feast.

I could not help comparing our Anglo-American graciousness, which is so full of reserve. Lavish display of food and affection is not appropriate and to give fully would be too embarrassing and intimate.

On my first visits to Abkhasian homes, I always assumed that the large number of people coming and going in connection with a feast were members of the immediate family. Actually, they were neighbors and relatives whose help is expected whenever a guest appears.

In the past, it was customary for the host to slaughter a ram for an overnight guest, even if there was already fresh meat in the house. Today, only the best grain, cheese, meat, and other products are used in feasting a guest. Even in cases of extreme poverty, the rules of hospitality are never violated, and a guest can expect to receive the family's last supplies, although he would probably not be aware of this. The guest, who may be only a stranger passing through, should not try to pay for his reception, since even a hint of an offer is considered a great insult. No matter how much one might want to avoid staying for dinner, one simply cannot do so without insulting the hosts, their families, their neighbors, and the entire village. When we visited and an invitation was extended, we had to remain, although we knew it would involve hours and hours of feasting and wine-drinking. The host who manages to keep his guests the longest and feed them to the limit of his resources is the one who is most admired.

Specific kinds of food served at feasts are discussed in greater detail in Chapter 6. Of course, the feast varies from region to region. In general, however, most feasts include *mamaligia* or bread, the ubiquitous cornmeal porridge, onions, cucumbers, tomatoes, garlic, cheese, roasted and boiled chicken, sauces and spices, boiled mutton, mutton on a spit, beef, fresh fruit, and nuts. Toasting the guest with wine throughout the meal is an important ritual in the Caucasus.

Wine is an integral part of a feast even in Moslem areas such as Abkhasia, Cherkessia, and Daghestan. Even in the orthodox Shiite region of Daghestan, in the past, wine was drunk at weddings; today Caucasian vodka is drunk on special occasions. In areas where the prohibition against alcohol was taken seriously, in Daghestan for example, a drink was made from grapes and stored in large clay vessels buried in the earth. My colleague Zyki Eglar, who studied the Moslem Cherkessians, found that their religious practice was restricted to the avoidance of pork and the celebration of two major religious holidays. "How can a Cherkessian live without wine?" she was asked when she inquired about the prohibition of alcohol. In these regions, wine is called "life-giving." The local physicians extoll its medicinal value, claiming that it prevents arteriosclerosis, for example. Since the wine is of low alcoholic content and is drunk more for the sake of toasting than anything else, even the very young and very old drink some with their meals, although everyone is expected to know his or her limits. When I showed surprise at seeing people drink wine without ever getting drunk, I was told, "With us, the dinner table is for oratory and toasting." In the Caucasus, where moderation in food and drink is the rule, it often seems that drinking is somewhat incidental to the social occasion. Since the Caucasians prefer lukewarm food, no one minds that the toasting and eating go on for hours with such deliberate decorum.

Custom dictates that immediately after sitting down, the eldest man present chooses a *tamada*, a toastmaster. The *tamada*, always a mature man, is the "ruler" or "prince" of the table. He determines the agenda of toasts and speeches and is privileged to drink two glasses of wine to everyone else's one. Legends are told of great *tamadas*, such as Sandro of Georgia, who had no occupation other than being invited to feasts and leading the toasts. The toast is a traditional poetic narrative, praising at great length the virtues, real or imagined, of each participant. In addition to toasting each guest, the *tamada* makes toasts on more general themes—toasts to love, to mothers, to those who are worse off, or to enemies. He must describe the person to whom the toast is proposed, and then speak lyrically of himself, his dreams and hopes, with many flowery, ornate comparisons. Each person in turn, regardless of rank or social position, is toasted to the evident delight of everyone. Only after the *tamada* has made all the major toasts will he select individuals to reply in thanks. With great flourish and eloquence, each guest stands up and makes a little speech thanking the *tamada*.

When a person is toasted he is supposed to wait until everyone else has finished drinking before he empties his own glass. Often a large horn with a silver rim is used for toasting. The wine is drunk in a single draught. When the toast is to important guests or their country, and so on, all present are exhorted to drain their glasses. During the long toasts, everyone listens without touching the glass.

Caucasians drink with decorum, enjoying their long toasts. When Caucasians drink, they do not cry or bare their souls. They are never profane. A festive dinner may last for three or four hours. No one may leave the table without the permission of the *tamada*. But if one has to leave, he cannot return to the table. The Georgians say of themselves: "We like to dance, sing, and drink."

The Caucasians are not only good narrators, but also patient listeners, in keeping with their rules of courtesy. When I was first called upon to make a speech at an Abkhasian banquet where about twenty-five people were present, I was unfamiliar with the structure of the toasts and was more nervous than I had ever been in front of a class of graduate students. The polite calm with which my hosts listened to my first fumbling attempt at Abkhasian eloquence showed not even the slightest hint of condescension or impatience.

Wherever I traveled in the Caucasus, my driver was always included in the feasting and toasting, although he was expected to observe greater than usual moderation in drink so as to be able to drive me home safely. Despite their concern with rank and deference, the Caucasians are a democratic people. Their deep democracy is clearly reflected in their toasting.

When parents are not at home, children are expected to act in their stead to entertain guests in the proper manner. Even a twelve-year-old boy should know the proper rituals for handwashing, seating arrangements, and toasting. The children, like the adults, love oratory and practice with each other. In the presence of elders, however, children are not supposed to be talkative.

The ritual of serving an honorary goblet *(nuazan)* is a characteristic feature of feasting in Ossetinia. Herodotus and ancient folk legends testify to the antiquity of this custom in the area. Describing the *nuazan,* Herodotus noted that after the Scythians had killed many of the enemy, the warriors would drink out of a special goblet. "But those who had not distinguished themselves could not touch this goblet. They sat on the side in great dishonor." In the Ossetinian Nart epic, this cup is called the *uatsamonga.* It would be filled with *rong* or beer and raised to the lips of those warriors who had distinguished themselves in battle. The *nuazan* custom was handed down from the Scythians, who were among the forebears of the Ossetinians and Cherkassians as well as the Kabardinians.

To this day, special rules are operative at the table when the honorary goblet is passed around. The person who receives the *nuazan* has the right to pass the goblet to anyone, with the permission of the eldest. In the past, among the plains Ossetinians, the guest did not have the right to leave until his host had given him the "guest goblet" to drink from.

The guest, too, has certain prescribed obligations. Just as neglecting to offer hospitality is considered immoral, rejecting hospitality is insulting. Indeed, in the villages, it was difficult for me to find graceful ways to avoid consuming two or three large meals in a row without giving offense. *Any meeting between two or more people can become the occasion for happy feasting, with full observance of the forms and rituals.

The village of Pasanauri was reported to have a number of longevous people whom I wished to interview. A friend of mine, whose family lived in the village, arranged to drive me and some other people there. After a long day of chatting, interviewing, and photographing, our party of five went to a small inn to eat. As soon as we sat down, it was clear to me that the first order of business must be to elect a *tamada*. We elected a man from the village who was with us. He ordered the food and wine, and while the waiter was setting the table, went to get a musician friend to fill our evening with music. We spent hours dining on delicious *shashlyk* (shishkebab), *khatchapuri* (cheese cake), meat dumplings, cucumbers, radishes, and a variety of greens and spicy sauces, to the accompaniment of lilting Georgian songs and a running commentary by the *tamada*. He regaled us with stories and anecdotes, each punctuated with a glass of fine Georgian wine.

After a few hours of merrymaking, we were about to go back to the city, which was quite a distance away over icy mountain roads. Our *tamada* then pointed out that we could not leave without meeting his family and suggested that we stop by for a few minutes. We walked to his house, which was nearby. As soon as we entered, I was overwhelmed by the fragrance of cooking, and the table that had been set. The whole family gathered to greet us warmly. I wildly considered falling into a faint rather than risk offending them by refusing their hospitality; instead, I went to the mother and explained how sincerely grateful we were and how terribly sorry not to be able to accept her kindness. I said that I was extremely tired and faced a long journey over slippery roads. I said that I must rise early to work. Again, I said how truly sorry I was and asked her to excuse me. She seemed to understand and then came up with an agreeable solution: we would take with us all the food that could be loaded into our car! And so we did. She added that we must stop at the home of a relative to pick up the *khatchapuri* that had been baked there rather than at her house because of some difficulty with her stove. At the relative's house, we were again offered wine and gracious welcome. We added the *khatchapuri* to our load and went on our way, with enough food for myself and a number of friends to last for several days.

These ancient traditions of hospitality, although still observed in the villages, have naturally become somewhat diluted in the cities. But adaptations of these customs and the deeply ingrained habits of courtesy and generosity to guests manifest themselves in many ways, even in the cities.

On my last visit to the city of Tbilisi in the spring of 1975, I arrived quite late at night. The porter carried my bags to the room and helped in getting me settled. When I offered a tip, he absolutely refused, saying that I was their guest and besides, "we" have plenty of money. "We" would seem to mean all Georgians. My tips were declined throughout Georgia. Each Georgian, bearing responsibility for the hospitality of his community—indeed, the whole country—would not think of neglecting to please a guest and make him feel welcome.

Ten years ago, after an international congress of anthropologists in Moscow, the American delegation took a short trip to Tbilisi. It was a hot day and we wanted some fruit. We found a market in a narrow side street where a group of farmers were selling watermelons. There were eight of us, but only I spoke Russian. We selected a medium-sized watermelon, asked for the price, and paid. I chatted with the farmers for a few minutes while my colleagues talked to each other in English. Hearing an unfamiliar language, the man who sold me the melon asked where we were from. I said we were from the United States. "Did you really come such a long way just to visit us?" "Yes," I replied. The farmers were delighted and kept repeating how proud they were that we had come so far, from the great country of America, just to visit them. They promptly took back the melon we had bought, replaced it with a much larger one, and returned our money, explaining that a guest does not pay. When we refused to accept the gift, the man picked up the melon and proceeded to lead the whole party back to the hotel in procession, carrying the melon as if it were a ceremonial offering. We had no choice but to accept and planned to return the next day with gifts for the farmers. As we parted, thanking them for their gift, we received a shower of blessings from them, such as, "Let your sickness come to me."

The next day we returned to the market but found no one. I was told that the farmers come to town only when they have something to sell, or whenever the spirit moves them.

In the evening we were given a banquet by the anthropologists from Tbilisi, and I told the story of the melon. Ten years later, in Tbilisi, I met a professor who had heard the story at that dinner. He told me that he tells it to every freshman class in Tbilisi to remind them that they must be alert to the presence of guests in their midst so that they could show them proper Georgian hospitality. I laughed and told him that I, too, tell this story to *my* students in New York as a fine example of Georgian hospitality and generosity.

Throughout the Caucasus, I met proud and generous people. I was given not only meals, but also gifts—countless packages of tea from their plantations, fruit, nuts, or some handwork. We tried not to let our interviewees know in advance when we were going to visit them, because no matter how poor they would be sure to prepare a meal for us.

When I was in Tbilisi, my assistant always managed to pay for tickets in advance, even when I had invited her. She was a lovely young Georgian woman, eager to exercise her English, so I took her along on my trips to take notes for me. One day I invited her for dinner in a fashionable restaurant. When I asked for the bill, the waiter told me that it had been paid by another guest—the director of the archeological museum who was in the restaurant at the time and recognized us. I was embarrassed, but my assistant assured me that it is a common courtesy for both men and women guests. I could not even thank the gentleman since he had already left.

In the summer of 1974 I had a dress altered in a government-run shop in Sukhumi. When I picked it up, the manager refused to accept payment, saying, "You are in Abkhasia. You are our guest!"

The day I left Sukhumi, my friends Dr. Inal-Ipa and his wife took me to a fine restaurant. Shortly after we sat down, bottles of wine began to arrive, sent to our table by friends of the Inal-Ipas'. Our table soon became too small to hold all the bottles, and one of our assistants organized a veritable "wine cellar" on the floor beside our table. In the meantime, word went around that Dr. Inal-Ipa was entertaining an American guest, and the orchestra leader announced an American song in my honor. I never recognized the melody, but was pleased by the intention. The waiter gave away the bottles we left. It is considered bad manners to take along the bottles not used.

All my efforts to reciprocate were overwhelmed by the generosity toward a guest which followed me everywhere in the Caucasus.

Why did these traditions of hospitality become so elaborate and ritualized? Feasting and entertaining are the basis of almost all social intercourse in the Caucasus, and a great many community functions are advanced at these gatherings. The physical isolation of mountain settlements made entertaining travelers and neighboring villagers absolutely essential for contact with other human beings. A transient bread-breaking was not enough to insure the permanence and continuity of these contacts, and so hospitality had to be invested with elaborate ceremony and the utmost generosity in order to solidify and perpetuate the relationships thus established. The security of a family or village depended on cementing friendships with other families and villages.

The absence of a central government and the division of the area into a number of fiercely independent groups may be another historical reason for the extreme stress on hospitality. Like the Greek city-states which made Zeus the god of guests to emphasize the importance of hospitality, the Caucasian peoples may have developed their ritualized rules of hospitality to guarantee the protection of the traveler far from home. A host was obliged to defend his guest to the death. In areas where there were many different peoples, each with its own language and customs and with no common legal code, hospitality guaranteed the traveler's rights and life despite the absence of a law-enforcement agency. To cement friendships between different families belonging to different lineages, host and guest often became ritual brothers. Every family extending hospitality to members of other families expected reciprocity from them. Hospitality thus became a social mechanism for providing people away from home with food, shelter, and safety.

Caucasian folklore, poetry, and even modern dramas are full of stories of selfless devotion to guests. Should a guest come without an invitation, he is automatically entitled to food, shelter, and protection for at least three days. In former times, a guest was to be protected not only by his host but by the entire community, no matter who was pursuing him or what he had done.

An Abkhasian folk story is told about a small rabbit being chased by hunters. He hid under the cloak of an old man attending a village meeting. The old man immediately pronounced the rabbit to be his guest and flatly refused to surrender him.

A much more painful version of this story is told in a modern Caucasian drama, which is performed often and illustrates the sacred obligation to protect a guest at no matter what cost. It also demonstrates the high value placed on self-restraint and discipline in the Caucasus. A young man bursts into a humble hut where an old man sits beside the fire, grief-stricken because he has received news that his son is dead. The young man begs for refuge because he is being pursued, and the old man finds him a hiding place in the house. Later, a group of men from the young man's lineage arrive and demand that the old man tell them whether he has seen the fugitive. He denies any knowledge, but they insist that he must be hiding him. The old man remains firm, even when he learns that the fugitive has killed his own son. Finally, the pursuers leave and the old man, still maintaining rigid control and superhuman restraint, sends his son's slayer quietly on his way with proper directions for an escape route through the mountains.

There is an Abkhasian legend about a robin who was busy arranging her nest when a guest arrived unexpectedly. She had nothing to offer him and in her anguish and shame, she cut her own breast open. Blood gushed out of the wound and stained her feathers. Touched by her sense of honor and hospitality, God decreed that she should live but have red feathers on her breast so that people would honor her. Abkhasian children, who often raid birds' nests, do not touch the robin redbreast's home.

A major prestige item in Caucasia was a separate guest house. When a son built a house next to his family's, all shared the large front lawn and the guest house. If the family did not have a separate guest house, a special room was usually set aside for the comfort and entertainment of guests.

Among some Caucasians, it was considered improper for the elder of the house or lineage to leave the guest alone for even a single hour. The guest slept in the special guest room. While the oldest guest was preparing for bed, all the remaining guests and hosts stood by his bed. The youngest guest or one of the host's sons took off the eldest guest's shoes and washed his feet. The footwear of other guests was also taken off for them but they had to wash their own feet. Usually the left shoe was taken off first; then the buttons on the *cherkeska* (coat) and *beshmet* (shirt) were undone from top to bottom. For dressing, the order of buttoning was reversed.

When the guest was leaving, the men accompanied him. The guest was never seated on his horse or cart in the presence of women. Holding his felt cloak, hat, and shawl in his left hand, a guest approached his horse. Then, transferring his things to his right hand and turning his horse's head toward the house, the guest mounted his horse, the eldest mounting first. After mounting, shaking hands was not permitted. The guest was not permitted to hit his horse in the vicinity of the house, lest the host think that the guest was somehow dissatisfied. The guest was accompanied to the outskirts of the village or even to his next stop. If a guest were insulted or killed, the host and his relatives were expected to avenge his honor or death.

In the Caucasus, the traditional friend or friendship relationship is called *kunak*. Not all *kunak* are the same, however. The most important *kunak* are those inherited from one's parents. They keep close ties with the family, helping in all ways, including financially when necessary. They must come to the protection of members of the family. The development of commerce made it almost a necessity for a man to have a *kunak* when traveling. A *kunak* or ritual friend automatically became the guest of all one's relatives who lived in the same village.

If a traveler had no relatives or *kunak* in a particular village, the head of the village assigned him to a certain lineage. In order to make the guest's time more pleasurable, musicians, dancers, and storytellers were invited to entertain him. The guest, even if a stranger, should never offer to pay but was expected to reciprocate if the opportunity arose.

One of the important virtues which all Caucasians share is the respect for etiquette. Etiquette for them is not a nicety which can be dismissed as superfluous but a basic structural design for living. Caucasians are friendly with the Russians, but they are sometimes disturbed by Russian informality.

Behavior between Caucasian friends is highly structured. The Russians believe that friends can set aside the conventions, but the Caucasians would do that only with an enemy.

When I commented to a Cherkessian emigré princess that her people are very formal in dealing with one another, she replied that this was simply a sign of mutual respect. The princess told me about a Kabardinian man who came to visit her in New York. He entered the room, crossed to the opposite side, and flopped himself down on the sofa while his hostess was still standing. She asked sympathetically whether he felt sick. Did he need a pillow? When he seemed surprised by the questions, she told him that she had never seen a Caucasian behave in this manner. Since the man was both younger than she and lower in rank, his behavior was especially surprising.

The princess also spoke about the casual way the Russians dismiss their partners at the end of a dance. She said that when she was young, at the end of a dance the partners backed away from each other, taking small steps until they were back in their pre-dance positions.

Informality is a sign that one is considered to be of a lower status and is taken as an insult. Even children and servants are treated with structured formality. The slightest insult is to be avoided at all costs. Any lack of observation of this strict etiquette is an affront to honor.

Children are drilled in good manners from the time they are very young. They are rebuked if they fall short of the standards of being "respectable," a word used constantly in correcting their behavior. Observance of the rules of etiquette is far more strict in the country than in the city. In both, however, a breach of etiquette is regarded as an insult, even between friends. To be rude is to disregard the other person's honor.

I was surprised to hear how often Caucasians use the Russian word *opozoritsia* (shame, disgrace). At first, I thought that a speaker with a limited Russian vocabulary might sometimes use stronger words than necessary. Later I realized how intentional the strong word is. An insult must never be forgotten. One should defend one's honor even if the opportunity for retaliation does not come for a long time.

The Caucasians believe that the observance of formal rules is the only guarantee against rudeness. The line between acceptable and unacceptable behavior is very sharply drawn. An outsider who does not know the rules of a culture feels, at the very least, highly uncomfortable. A native who violates these rules may find himself in mortal danger. There is a saying: "There is nothing that a Caucasian would not do for a friend and nothing that he would not do to an enemy." Acceptance and hospitality are always initially assumed in the Caucasus, unlike many other cultures; violation of this presumed friendship is dealt with by a dagger. A statue in Tbilisi, symbolizing Georgia, has a cup of wine in one hand for friends and a sword in the other hand for enemies.

I violated the cultural norms at the beginning of my field work in Abkhasia. I asked for permission to visit a village household, but the time was not specified and I was not invited for dinner. I brought with me a box of chocolates as a gift. The hostess disappeared immediately to prepare food. It was assumed that I would stay for dinner. The host, who had come out to greet me, accepted the gift with some embarrassment. He expected to give a gift, not receive one—as I later learned. Nothing was said about my mistake, but upon leaving I found several pounds of tea in my car. This gift was from my host's share of the tea grown on his collective farm and had been part of his payment. It is considered that a guest bestows an honor by visiting and the gift is a token of the host's gratitude.

Gift-giving is a very important part of the social life of the Caucasus. Very often, one must give away something simply because it is praised or desired by someone else. From early childhood, one must learn to be able to give up even the most precious possession without regret. Perhaps this is why the Caucasians never developed a great emotional attachment for things, except perhaps for their horses—but horses were not merely possessions, but often were necessary for their very lives.

Gift-giving does not depend on the social hierarchy but, as in a great many other cultures, is used to establish friendships and loyalty. A Georgian friend commented, "Gift-giving in the U.S. is a comedy. After the Christmas season, people rush back to the department stores to exchange their gifts for something else. If the sales check is included, they try to get the money. Our gift-giving is of a different nature. We give gifts freely. We do not exchange gifts for other items or for money." When someone comes for dinner or for a short stay with a Georgian family, he may bring some flowers, but not a real gift. However, it is customary for the host to give the guest a gift as a remembrance of the visit. Any personal possession may be given as a gift.

A friend of mine visited a Georgian home in New York. Forgetting the custom that the Russians used to call *pesh-kesh* (what's mine is yours), she admired a chandelier in the sitting room and said that it was of the type she had wanted for her study. The Georgian hostess had the chandelier taken down and sent it to my friend, who protested without success.

Gift-giving brings honor and a feeling of satisfaction to the giver. It also demonstrates the honored position of the guest. A man feels that by giving he elevates himself in his own eyes and shows others and himself that he can afford it. The most important thing is the increase in self-esteem. When a man intends to give a gift to a guest whom he likes, he tries in a very roundabout way to find out whether the guest likes anything in particular among his possessions. Then, on parting, he hands the gift to the guest, so that the guest is not embarrassed by having praised something openly and then receiving it as a gift. There is a Georgian saying: "You like it, take it." An Abkhasian proverb states, "What you withhold from a good friend will bring you no pleasure."

5
FOLK MEDICINE

Even in ancient times, the Caucasian people were known to have a highly developed folk medicine. Horace and Dioscoridus (first century, B.C.) and Ammian Marcellinus (fourth century, A.D.) all mention the preparation of medications by the Kolkhidians and Iberians, ancient Georgian tribes. The Roman naturalist, Pliny the Elder, writing in the first century A.D., noted that various medicines were imported into the Mediterranean region from Armenia.

The medical skill of the Georgian tribes is mentioned in the myths of the ancient Greeks, who traded with them for medicines and plants. Gekat and Medea, the wife and daughter of Aeëtes, the mythical king of Colchis (Kolkhida, or present-day Georgia), are described in the Argonaut myth as being skillful pharmacists. Medea's artistry with narcotics and poisons is especially well-known. She presented Jason with a robe soaked in poison in revenge for deserting her and their two children.

Hippocrates (460–377 B.C.), the "father of medicine," was supposed to have visited Kolkhida. He was highly impressed by the healthful diet, the lean, strong physiques, the beauty, the customs, and especially the hospitality of the Caucasian people. As early as the first century B.C., the Greek scholar Dioscorides named many of the plants still common today in his work on Caucasian herbs.

The *Karabadini,* medieval Georgian medical books, contain a wealth of data collected by observation and experience through the centuries. With the introduction of Christianity into Georgia in the fifth century, elements of mysticism appeared in the folk medicine. The clergy managed to fuse mysticism and religious ritual with the practical knowledge of folk medicine. A typical ritual for a sick person, for example, might begin with praise for the deity of the disease; then, the symptoms of the disease were described in imagery, followed by a listing of the medical treatments for the disease, and finally the deity of the disease was praised once again. (The folk doctors, however, continued to enjoy greater popularity than the religious healers. People believed, pragmatically, that if it was possible to diagnose and treat a disease initially, it was not necessary to seek help from the deities.) Georgians and Abkhasians believed that every epidemic had a special angel or master who brought it, and who stayed with the sick person. One had to try to please them, or they would never leave without exacting human life. The sickroom was decorated in bright colors and the angel was entertained with special songs which lulled it to sleep.

In the Caucasus, there are over 550 varieties of wild-growing medicinal plants which continue to be used in folk medicine today. Many of them, now also used throughout the world by modern medicine, have retained their Caucasian names. Several contemporary medical procedures in the Soviet Union and elsewhere—such as the use of hot mud, sea baths, and changes of climate—have their origin in Caucasian folk medicine.

Various methods of refining raw materials were used in the preparation of medicines. Both open and hermetically sealed vessels were used to prepare broths of leaves and grasses. Ground-up plants were often brewed in milk, wine, or water and kept in special vessels made of wood, clay, or wax. The gathering of each medicinal plant involved a special ritual at a particular time of the year. A precise methodology evolved which dictated not only the proper time for harvesting, but also the parts of the plants—leaves, stems, roots—to be used for specific diseases as well as the form of the preparation —liquid exudate, powder, or the leaves themselves.

A medical inventory, published at the beginning of the nineteenth century and far from complete, listed 569 medications known in Georgia, 372 of which were prepared from plants, fifty-five from animal substances, thirty from minerals, seventeen from precious stones, and ninety-five of mixed composition. Along with the stalks, roots, leaves, and fruits of plants, this work lists animal organs, honey, wine, salt, potash, lime, and flint as common medicinal substances. Bear and goat fat, vegetable oils, and potash were the primary base substances for administering the medicine.

Folk doctors who treated open wounds, fractures, severe bruises, and so forth enjoyed special respect throughout the Caucasus since they were very successful. The most skilled doctors of the Khevsuretia and Svan tribes in the mountain regions of Georgia could perform abdominal operations and trepanations of the skull. Daghestanians were known as specialists in circumcision. Since the demand was and still is great, and the number of trained folk doctors is limited, some groups of Moslems often have to wait several years for the arrival of a doctor. As a result, not all boys were circumcised by the accepted age of four years. In tradition-minded families, folk doctors still perform circumcisions. Other folk doctors specialized in removing gallstones. The removal of cataracts, also performed by other ancient Eastern peoples, was successfully practiced.

Although these doctors' conceptions were often primitive, their understanding of anatomy was quite advanced. Surgical techniques and procedures were meticulously worked out, although the instruments were often very simple. Trepanation is still done by folk doctors in remote villages, but now they use antibiotics as well.

Modern Soviet medicine believes that Georgian folk doctors were the first to use dried blood to stop bleeding. This method, widely used in mountainous Georgia, was described in a Georgian medical book of the eleventh century, and remains in use today.

In Daghestan, folk surgery developed into an even more sophisticated science than in Georgia. In his *History of the War and Russian Control in the Caucasus* (St. Petersburg, 1871), N. Dubrovin writes:

The results of surgical operations are simply unbelievable. There is not a single kind of wound, with the exception of mortal injuries, which the local surgeons are not able to cure without ill aftereffects to the patient. Neither the season of year, nor temperature, seems to affect him—no nausea or pain during or before the onset of bad weather is felt.

Amputation was performed quickly, using a simple knife, with minimal pain: there were rarely ill consequences. The amputee rarely or never died and never under the knife of the surgeon.

Daghestanian folk doctors were trained either in their families or by other folk doctors. The skills were gathered empirically and handed down from generation to generation. Anyone with interest and ability could become a doctor. It was a matter of finding a willing teacher. The same is true today. Although now each village or group of villages has a modern doctor and some kind of medical field unit, nevertheless many people use the folk doctors and go to the others only if they do not improve.

Another Russian scholar, N.I. Pirogov, writes at the end of the nineteenth century of the Daghestanians' "great experience and skill in treating wounds from firearms." The art of curing external wounds, passed down from father to son, was a skill forced upon the mountain people by the exigencies of war. Wounds made by firearms and steel weapons advanced the development of folk surgery. During the Caucasian War in the nineteenth century, many contemporaries praised the competence of the Daghestanians in healing wounds, fractures, and severe bruises. A Lieutenant Runovskij, who served in the Russian army, writes that their cures "could seem unbelievable, if there hadn't been so many people, healed by these surgeons, who serve as living evidence of their skill."

Bleeding was stopped effectively by Daghestanian folk doctors. A little salt would be sprinkled on the wound, and then it would be bound with a tourniquet. Although the salt could have had little effect as a disinfectant, it may have contributed to the upkeep of general body tone, an important factor in serious injuries. Also, singed sheep wool was used. It was found to stop bleeding much faster than spider web—which is a bactericide much like the mold from which we now get penicillin.

The *khakim* or mountain folk doctors practiced blood-letting. Leeches were first put into a dish of water and then placed on the "suffering part of the body" until they were engorged with blood and fell off.

Daghestanian folk doctors prepared medicine for ailing joints, rheumatism, and even cholera. Broths of grasses, taken internally, and ointments were used quite successfully for rheumatism but internal diseases in general presented great difficulties to the folk doctor. There were no effective cures until modern times.

Smallpox, which decimated and scarred whole generations of mountain people, was a terrible scourge in Daghestan. Despite their proximity to Russian settlements, most Daghestanians knew nothing about vaccination, and those who had heard of it did not tend to believe in its worth.

In Georgia and other areas of the Caucasus, however, vaccination against smallpox was practiced even in ancient times by specialist folk doctors who prepared the vaccine from the pus of persons afflicted with a mild form of smallpox. Without modern immunological theories, they nevertheless understood that mild forms of the disease could bestow immunity against the more virulent forms. Before Jenner's cowpox method, children were deliberately exposed to the milder forms of smallpox. The shirt of a mildly sick child, for example, would be put on a healthy child.

Since all contagious diseases, especially smallpox, were thought to come from angels, the folk doctors frequently resorted to certain rituals. In the sickroom, absolute cleanliness and silence were maintained. The silence was broken on ritual occasions when songs praising the "angels of the disease" were sung to the accompaniment of a harp. Of course these rituals were neither Christian nor Moslem, for in the early days of Christianity all kinds of pagan rites were incorporated. Even now, some of the old people still practice these rites without giving a thought to whether they are Moslem or Christian, simply because they are part of the tradition.

In the Soviet Union, folk medicine has now become the object of special pharmaceutical and clinical study. The ancient medical treatments, derived from empirical observation and verified by long experience, are being prescribed throughout the Soviet Union, although a network of modern clinics has been established.

The elderly, especially, are the guardians of the ancient lore. The Caucasus, as I have said, is very rich in wild-growing medicinal plants. The majority of old people know where these plants can be found and how to prepare medications. During the spring and summer, many long-living individuals prepare large supplies of medicinal plants for their own needs and to sell to pharmacists.

The plants used as medicines by the longevous are not intended simply to treat a specific ailment. A whole group of food plants are considered to have not only nutritional but also medicinal properties and are used both to treat and to prevent disease. Therapeutic and preventive medicine are part of a more general concept of health as the "normal" state of being, with longevity as the natural outcome of a healthy life. The functions of food in health and illness are carefully prescribed.

In most Caucasian folk medicine, especially Georgian, great attention is given to diet. A Georgian medicinal book of the eleventh century says:

Most sicknesses are intensified by food. A small sickness can develop into a large one, depending on what the sick person eats. The doctor should prescribe the diet along with medication. The important thing is that a sick person should eat very light food.

It also mentions that abstinence from food or semi-hunger is beneficial. And

if one has high blood pressure, he should eat cold, sour foods, because this clears the blood and lowers the pressure. When someone has gallstones, he should abstain from meat and, as for fruit, he should eat only pomegranates and apples.

It suggests that if one cannot walk or work, he should cook meat until it is almost liquefied in order to be able to digest it. "In the case of hemorrhoids, one should not eat onions, peppers, or garlic. If one has varicose veins, one should not eat food that is difficult to digest." Indigestible food may cause constipation, which aggravates varicose veins and hemorrhoids.* In mental illness, meat is forbidden, but fruits such as pomegranates, apples, and pears are acceptable.

Honey is a good example of a food with both nutritional and medicinal value. It is called the "sweet medicine," and, like wine, it has been used from time immemorial in the Caucasus as a medication for colds and related complaints. It is drunk in warm milk or lemon juice, or made into a syrup with horseradish.† It is used to treat gastritis and ulcers, since it normalizes the acidity of the stomach and facilitates the functioning of the bowels. By increasing glycogen in the liver, it aids hydrocarbon exchange and protein, fat, vitamin, and hormone metabolism, thus raising the level of resistance to infections. Since ancient times honey has been considered an excellent sedative and tranquilizer.

It has been used by Soviet doctors for the treatment of diseases of the eye, especially for burns on the eye. It is used in the treatment of certain skin diseases. It is heated and its vapors are inhaled for infections of the upper respiratory system. Honey is also recommended for stomach and heart trouble.

The presence in honey of over eighty substances important for the human organism, such as glucose, many trace elements, fermentation products, organic acids, minerals, hormones, antibiotics, and pollen (in itself a source of substances important for the organism) gives honey both its nutritional and therapeutic values. Dr. M. Sultanov, a noted Soviet gerontologist and a great advocate of the therapeutic value of honey, recommends it especially for the very young and very old. No more than a quarter of a cup of honey should be taken daily, preferably in two or three dosages, two or three hours before and after meals.

Honey has been and still is widely used for cosmetic purposes by Caucasian women. It is warmed and spread over the face, where it is thought to pene-

---

*Many American doctors believe that our refined, high-carbohydrate diet is an important etiologic factor in hemorrhoids, cancer of the colon, colitis, appendicitis, and possibly varicose veins because of decreased stool bulk, constipation, and increased stool-transit time.

†Lime blossom honey is used in tea for colds in Abkhasia. This variety of honey, also considered useful in the treatment of diarrhea, derives its medicinal value from the lime tree itself, the bark of which is made into a porridge with milk to make compresses for infected wounds.

trate the skin, nourishing and softening it. Honey with crushed almonds is still used as a facial mask at night to prevent wrinkles.

Some of the uses of honey in folk medicine in the United States are surprisingly similar to those used in the Caucasus. Dr. D.C. Jarvis, in his well-known book *Folk Medicine,* discusses old folk remedies in Vermont and devotes twenty-four pages to the curative properties of honey. The minerals present in honey are enumerated: iron, copper, manganese, silica, chlorine, calcium, potassium, sodium, phosphorus, aluminum, and magnesium. He also credits honey with very high vitamin C content.

The Vermont folk, as well as the Caucasians, believe that a teaspoon of honey taken before bedtime induces sleep. It is also used by people in both areas as a cough medicine when mixed with some milk, and as a relief for leg and feet muscle cramps when taken at each meal.

Garlic *(Allium sativum)* seems to be one of the oldest plants used by people. The Egyptians are said to have given garlic to the pyramid-builders to protect them against disease. In the Middle East, garlic was used to prevent sexual impotence. Garlic is useful for lowering blood pressure, combating bacteria, and relieving rheumatism. It has vitamins A, C, B_1, and B_2. It is another common food which is considered beneficial for health everywhere in the Caucasus. In Abkhasia it is used to cure a very bad cold. A pound of garlic is put through a grinder (or it may be crushed by hand) and added to one pint of ninety-six-proof vodka. The bottle is covered with black paper to shield it from light and allowed to stand for ten days. To dispel the odor while preparing this recipe, a few leaves of mint can be added. The mixture is then strained through cheesecloth and allowed to stand for another three days. It is then ready for use. A drop is added to a small amount of milk and taken three times a day. The antibiotics found in garlic are highly effective against a variety of microorganisms, including dysentery and plague microbes. The well-known Abkhasian doctor, Dr. Kakiashvili, told me of a folk remedy to prevent calcification of the bones and around the joints using this mixture of garlic and vodka. In the days of cholera epidemics, people hung crushed garlic cloves in little bags around their necks in the belief that its strong odor and curative properties would prevent infection.

A mustard poultice is used as a rubefacient to improve the local flow of blood. Mustard is used not only as a spice but is also mixed in water to soak tired legs.

Barberry *(Oxyacantha)* is a versatile plant used in both folk medicine and cooking. It is a treelike shrub about thirteen feet high with a brownish-purple stem and thorns about an inch and a half long. It produces a small, oval berrylike blood-red fruit which is collected just before it ripens in September. The young leaves are a common substitute for sorrel; the fruit, both fresh and dried, is used in soups for its sour flavor. Syrup, jam, and marmalade are prepared from the soft parts of the ripe fruit in place of lemon. The fruits, blossoms, and root bark are used medicinally. Barberry is thought to improve the appetite and strengthen heart muscles. In some areas, it is used to treat bleeding, diarrhea, rheumatism, fever, edema, and diseases of the eyes and mouth. The berries are dried in the sun or in a warm place. When fully dried, they should be dark red. Black ones are discarded. The dried berries are stored in boxes in a dry place, since they absorb moisture easily. They are effective in treating digestive disorders, gall stones, or difficulties in urination. They are very high in vitamin C. One teaspoonful of the berries is added to a cup of boiling water, covered, allowed to steep for about ten minutes, strained, and drunk once daily before eating. This brew reduces nervous tension and increases blood circulation in the vessels of the heart and brain. According to Dr. Kakiashvili, a prominent Abkhasian physician, it was tested in the treatment of experimentally induced arteriosclerosis in rabbits. The results indicated that the *Oxyacantha* extract reduces the amount of lipids on the walls of the arteries, reducing arterial pressure and relieving blood-vessel spasms.

Tea made from certain apples *(Malus domesticata Borkh)* is used for gall stones, rheumatism, coughing, and chronic stomach problems.

Modern Soviet medicine has found that *Citrulus Pang,* a melon used widely in folk medicine, is rich in carotene, ascorbic acid, nicotinic acid, and vitamins B_1 and B_2.

Garden dill *(Anethum graveolens)* is used widely as a cathartic and diuretic and for hypertension and stomach-aches as well as in food. The seeds contain a mixture of terpines and volatile oil. The leaves contain ascorbic acid, carotene, and the anticoagulant warfarin. Tea is brewed from the leaves and taken internally. There is evidence that the drinking of dill tea may lower arterial pressure, widen the arterial passages, and stimulate the heart. It is being used by the Soviet medical profession in the treatment of high blood pressure. Dill also acts as an anti-flatulant. A teaspoonful of ground dill seeds is added to one and a half cups of boiling water. This mixture is cooled, strained, and taken in half-glass doses three times a day on an empty stomach.

A tea made from marjoram leaves is thought to relieve muscle spasms.

Sage, *(Salvia)* is a flavoring herb to which some old people attribute their longevity. It is the legendary herb of wisdom and immortality. Brewed as a tea, it is used as a gargle for sore throats.

Tarragon, still used in the Caucasus, was employed by the early Arabian physician Avicenna (980–1037 A.D.) for medicinal purposes.

Thyme *(Thymus vulgaris)* is believed to be good for the nervous system and is brewed in tea.

Yarrow *(Achillea milletolium)* is capable of agglutinating blood. A friend of mine tried it on herself and found that it readily stops bleeding. It is also called *Meliscuda,* little fox tail.

There are, of course, plants used exclusively as medicines in the Caucasus. I brought back a number of dried medicinal plants that had been identified by Soviet pharmacists. The descriptions and uses of these plants were collected in interviews with physicians and native informants.

The dogrose or doghip sweetbriar *(Rosa canina)* is used very widely not only in folk medicine but also by the pharmaceutical industry in the preparation of chologogues, substances which stimulate the output of bile by the liver. The fruit of the dogrose, rich in provitamin A (carotene), ascorbic acid (vitamin C), riboflavin (vitamin B₂), citrin (vitamin R), and vitamin K, are used in the treatment of hepatitis and inflammation of the gall bladder. Tea made from the fruit is used against tuberculosis, infectious diseases, inflammation of the liver and gall bladder, ulcers, and chronic stomach trouble. The red, round berries (not the elongated, dark berries) are boiled in a pint of water and allowed to stand overnight. This tea is drunk twice a day in one-glass dosages.

Motherwort *(Leonorus cardiaca),* a member of the mint family, is native to the Caucasus and has been used by the people there for a very long time. During the last few years it has become a very popular herb sold in drugstores throughout the Soviet Union. Harvested between June and September, it contains alkaloids, glucose, volatile oils, ascorbic acid, and vitamin A. It is not toxic. It is used to quiet the central nervous system, to relieve stomach gas, and to aid digestion. The preparation is simple. Three ounces of dried motherwort (excluding the stem) are added to boiling water and boiled for fifteen minutes. The tea is then strained and taken internally, one tablespoonful three to six times a day.

The leaves of *Plantago Major* are used to prepare a tea for the treatment of malaria and bladder infections. One to one-and-a-half teaspoons of dried leaves are steeped in a cup of boiling water. The mixture is strained and taken five or six times a day.

Malaria is treated with *Ranunculi,* a member of the buttercup family.

Another common plant, *Poligonaceae,* a bright-red-flowered member of the buckwheat family, is used as an anticoagulant and for treating colds. In buckwheat, researchers have found a substance known in our country as coumadin, a potent remedy for embolic and thrombotic occlusions, thus proving that the Caucasians were right to use the plant as an anticoagulant.

The roots of *Dioscorea caucasica* are used to make an extract, *Diosponium,* which reduces the cholesterol content of the blood and lowers arterial pressure. In the Soviet Union, *Diosponium* is used in the treatment of arteriosclerotic cerebral vascular and coronary artery disease. It is interesting to note that the root of the wild yam *(Dioscorea panicula,* closely related to *Dioscorea caucasica)* is used in the treatment of rheumatism. In the early stages of what was to be research on cortisone, the wild yam was substituted for animal adrenal glands.

Coriander *(Coriandrum sativum)* is one of the oldest plants used by man for food and medicinally. A teaspoon of seeds are steeped in one cup of boiling water, covered and left to stand for twenty minutes, and then strained. Two tablespoonsful three times daily are supposed to regulate the digestive process, prevent muscular spasms, and assist the liver and gall bladder.

The valerian plant *(Valeriana officinalis)* is used as a relaxant. Medicinally, only the roots are utilized. It is used to ease pain and relieve extreme nervous exhaustion and hysterical conditions. One tablespoon of the roots, combined with one cup of boiling water, is left to stand covered for fifteen minutes, then strained. The entire cup is then drunk in small doses. It should not be taken continuously for a period of time because it can affect digestion.

Phytotherapy, a technique developed by the staff of the Health Center (Zona Zdorovya) in Baku, is based on breathing the scents of special potted plants grown in an experimental greenhouse. The rationale of the "plant therapy" is that the nerve endings in the nasal cavity affect most of the organs of the body.

Scents can be divided into beneficial or deleterious, simple or complex, and organic or inorganic. Plant scents are organic. The power of a scent and indeed the scent itself depend on the chemical mixture. Laurel, pelargonium, santonin, and rosemary are all plants with curative scents. The biologically active volatile substances which they give off have a beneficial effect on the organism. The staff of the Zona Zdorovya and their followers believe that this treatment is especially effective for insomnia and diseases of the respiratory and circulatory systems. The director, Professor S. M. Gusanov, writes:

Curative plants such as beneficial laurel and rosemary contain negatively charged ions that bring about a beneficial action on the body, especially for such illnesses as nerve disorders and diseases of the cardio-vascular system.

It is possible that phytotherapy as a technique grew out of folk medicine, since folk medicine utilizes almost all of the medicinal plants of the Caucasus.

THERAPEUTIC USE OF MUSIC

Throughout the Caucasus music is used in folk medicine to relieve pain and as a tranquilizer. Each malady has its own specific song. Among the Kabardinians, Georgians, Armenians, Shapsugs, Balkars, and Abkhasians, "Songs of the Wounded" are sung to the accompaniment of a stringed instrument. One song is sung during the removal of a bullet, another during the dressing of the wound. Another song is sung to the wounded after the operation. There is a song which the wounded man's relatives, gathered around his bed, sing to him. The wounded man himself would sing "Songs of the Wounded" after he had been struck by a bullet on the field of battle, to tranquilize himself and reduce the pain.

Group singing is also used for illnesses. Neighbors and relatives spend the entire night at the bedside, playing stringed instruments, singing, dancing, and telling fairy tales, to distract the patient from his sufferings. The songs were considered holy; diseases were believed to have been sent by God, and the songs were sung not only to distract the sick person but also to "coax God" into curing him. This custom is still widespread in the Caucasus.

Music was also used as a psychological stimulus. Among the Abkasians a musician playing a stringed instrument, the *apkh'artsa,* would lead warriors into battle. The song "How to Get Down Someone Stuck in a Tree" was supposed to calm a person climbing down from a tree. In addition, music was used at funerals, wakes, and at the bedside of the dead. Because of the avoidance patterns between father and son, universal in the Caucasus, the father did not have the right to bemoan the loss of his son; singing was the only permitted expression of his woe.

Thus we see that in the Caucasus, medicine is not viewed as simply treatment of illness. Therapeutic and preventive medicine and nutrition are thought of as components of a healthy life. Medicines and foods are often interchangeable since the goal of both— a long and healthful life—is the same.

Dr. E. Grey Dimond, a prominent American physician, has commented that the emphasis on synthesized medicine since World War I "has left the West with little background to accept botanical remedies."

A great problem in describing folk medicine is that the quantities of various ingredients used are not given precisely. They seem to be based on individual experience. It might be compared to cooking before standard measurements were developed. This problem is particularly important when dealing with plants that are poisonous, since just a bit too much would produce an effect exactly opposite to the one intended.

My friend, Victor Geduldick, a pharmacist, wrote me a note after reading this chapter. He said:

In the age of steroids, heart transplants, and silicone breasts, folk medicine still has its place in curing illness as it had in the days of offerings and invocations to the deities that crowded the narrow world of our ancestors.

6

DO THEY ALL
EAT YOGURT?
NUTRITION
AND LONGEVITY

THE DIET

Of all the factors affecting the human body, diet is one of the most important. Many leading Soviet researchers regard diet as a determining factor in optimal development and adaptation to the environment. Diet, in great measure, also determines the length of useful physical activity. The character of the diet is of great importance for the general condition of the blood vessels, neural and hormonal systems, and metabolism.

Since diet is a particularly important factor in longevity, I devoted much time to investigating the food habits of long-living people and their families. This involved compiling data on food production, processing, and preparation for consumption. I encountered very firm beliefs about which foods should or should not be eaten to maintain good health.

There have been hundreds of observations and experiments done on animals and by people in many scientific communities, in an effort to establish dietary cause-and-effect in health and longevity. So far, no conclusive results have emerged, and efforts to correlate human diet and health are risky and difficult. One reason, of course, is that human beings, although members of the animal world, behave according to their cultural patterns, and not purely instinctually. Enormous complexity enters the question of nutrition and health because of the variety of cultural patterns around the world. It may be useful, however, to study human eating patterns within a specific society in which individuals are known to be longevous and to remain in good health.

Diet in the Caucasus has been stable for centuries, and remains so despite modern innovations. The introduction of new foods has brought only minor alterations, not essential changes. The use of traditional foods in a stable environment over many generations may produce a biological adjustment in man, allowing the organism to become accustomed to familiar foods. A regular dietary rhythm combined with a consistent, unchanging diet may reduce physiological stress on the organism, at least on the digestive system.

In the United States, and the industrial West in general, new foods are welcomed for their novelty. Eating patterns change drastically according to current nutritional theories, advertising campaigns, or marketing practices. The chaotic and inconsistent eating patterns of most Americans bring about diet-linked illnesses such as heart disease, diabetes, dysfunctions of the kidney, liver, and gall bladder, and, of course, obesity. Biologists often disagree with each other, but the connections between cardio-vascular disease and fat consumption, diabetes and sugar-intake, and so on are established. It will be a long time before precise causal relationships can be worked out, but no one, I think, can now deny the profound connection between diet and most of the diseases which afflict humans and consequently affect their longevity.

Dr. Samuel Rosen of Mount Sinai School of Medicine, New York, and his Soviet colleagues conducted a comparative epidemiological study of hearing in Moscow and in Abkhasia and Georgia. These studies confirmed the previous findings by Dr. Rosen about the effects of certain diets on hearing. Populations consuming large amounts of saturated fat do not seem to hear as well as those consuming smaller amounts of saturated fat combined with larger amounts of unsaturated fats. After testing the hearing in Abkhasia, Georgia, and Moscow, Dr. Rosen concluded that the significantly better hearing in Abkhasia and Georgia cannot be attributed to heredity, since the children in both areas, when tested, showed no difference in hearing, but rather to their diet, which has small amounts of saturated fats and large quantities of vegetables and fruit.

These culturally held beliefs about diet are worth describing, not only because at many points they coincide markedly with modern scientific knowledge, but also because they have produced a group of extraordinarily healthy and long-lived people.

Caucasian ethnic groups with longevous populations vary widely in ecological setting, religious belief, and degree of industrialization. All three factors influence the choice of food grown and used. The Moslems of Azerbaijan, Abkhasia, and Daghestan eat mostly mutton, some beef, but no pork. The Daghestanian and Azerbaijanian religion prohibits alcohol but some people drink a very light wine—in moderation. I found contrasting patterns of fat consumption—saturated, monounsaturated, and polyunsaturated. The consumption of sugar, vegetables, and milk products also varies widely.

Armenians eat eggs, but never in the evening as they consider eggs hard to digest.

Among all Caucasian peoples, the most ubiquitous milk product is *matzoni*, a cultured milk, similar in appearance and taste to yogurt. It has high food value and possesses therapeutic properties as well, especially for intestinal disorders. Because the action of lactic acid produces millions of living bacteria, yogurt has demonstrated antiseptic power. In the U.S., yogurt is recommended by physicians for patients whose intestinal flora have been temporarily wiped out—by taking antibiotics, for instance.

Despite many local variations in the Caucasus, certain general principles governing eating habits are, nevertheless, surprisingly uniform: rhythmic regularity in meals, an aversion to overeating, a calm, structured atmosphere at meals, absolute freshness of food. The close association of health and food in people's minds is universal throughout the Caucasus.

Fresh food, as far as we know, has been appreciated in both preliterate and modern Caucasian cultures. They do use dried meat when fresh is not available, and some pickled foods. Leftovers are discarded. They are aware that the loss of freshness means the loss of nutrients and good taste. The Caucasians consider storing unclean and unhealthy. Spices are ground just before they are used, and Caucasians avoid storing herbs, which gradually lose their flavor and color.

Wild-growing plants are plentiful in the woods and meadows of the Caucasus and are collected eagerly. They are equal if not superior to the cultivated species in vitamins, oils, protein, and natural sugars.

The wild nuts of the area contain 40 to 60 per cent oil, and some contain up to 20 per cent protein. The wild apples are sour and are very rich in vitamin C. Wild pears are also rich in vitamin C.

THE RULES OF DIET

Two factors remain constant in the Caucasian diet:

1. *No overeating.* Fewer calories are consumed in all areas of the Caucasus than the AMA recommends for Americans. Experiments conducted at Cornell University by Clive McKay showed that restricting caloric intake prolongs the life of rats, but only in the early period of life. A similar stretching out of earlier life was achieved by Denham Harman of the University of Nebraska.

2. *An extremely high intake of natural vitamins in fresh vegetables, both cultivated and wild.* They replace meat and sweet foods in the diet of the

Caucasians. This massive vitamin C intake could immunize the organism against many diseases.

Taking meals at a definite time, three or four times a day, is thought to develop a rhythm in the body. The most eminent Caucasian doctors cite irregular eating as a cause of stomach disorders. This belief in regularity is not restricted to diet but permeates the whole Caucasian life-style. In Moslem areas, lunch is eaten after the noontime prayer, which itself is performed regularly each day. Going to bed at night, rising in the morning, and taking meals are all factors in the development of a regular body rhythm.

Food is taken in very small bites and chewed thoroughly. Eating fast is considered boorish and unhealthy. A Cherkessian friend of mine recalled from her childhood that when children were sent visiting, they were fed at home before the journey so that they would not eat too fast on arrival. All Caucasians think of mealtime as relaxed and pleasurable. Meals often last several hours when guests are present. While the Abkhasians enjoy the music of the two-stringed *abkhartsa* during meals, the Azerbaijanian physician, M. Sultanov, recommends quiet music, and discourages youngsters and intellectuals from reading at mealtime! He claims that the attention reading requires diverts nervous impulses from the digestive glands. Telling sad stories at the table is considered bad manners. Festive occasions do not mean a change in the kinds of foods served and the atmosphere created, but rather the same ideas reign: freshness of food, moderation in eating, and a relaxed, even rhythm.

These rules of health and decorum are quite unbreakable and can create awkward moments for those who were not traditionally reared, as illustrated by the following story, told me by a Georgian woman who is now head of the Gerontological Institute of Tbilisi. City-reared in a family of intellectuals, she married a traditional Georgian at the age of seventeen. On her wedding day excitement and tension had kept her from eating for the entire day. When the wedding feast was served, she began to eat quickly and heartily. Her mother-in-law drew her gently away from the table and told her that one cannot eat so eagerly at the table. If she was that hungry, she should have a snack in the next room so that she could return to the feast and eat in the proper way—easily and slowly.

Throughout the Caucasus, a lean somatotype for both men and women is considered ideal. The obese person is considered ill. All of the Caucasian peoples have proverbs and sayings emphasizing the importance of moderation in eating. The Georgians consider that a man should be able to "eat at nine different tables," the Chechens pride themselves on never eating "the last spoonful," and the Azerbaijanian long-lived claim that they eat only enough to satisfy their hunger.

THE FAMILY HEARTH

Eating brings all the members of a large Caucasian family together. The hearth or wood-burning cookstove symbolized family unity. An enormous iron pot is suspended on a heavy chain over the stove—which in modern buildings may burn gas. All food is prepared in this kitchen, even if the extended family includes fifty or more.

Both the hearth and the chain above it were considered sacred by many Caucasian groups. A man took an oath by placing his right hand on the family chain. Evil fortune would come to the house if the chain was stolen. When the cooking pot becomes too small to feed the entire family, the oldest son, his wife, and children may build themselves a new home next to the father's. It is said by the Abkhasians that such a family has "broken its chain." The Cherkessians also place great significance on the chain and describe the extended family as "those who eat from the same cauldron" or "those who share a single chain over the fireplace." In Ossetia, the widow of the last male of a once-large family wears the kettle chain around her neck or waist while accompanying her husband's body to the graveyard. "May you wear a kettle chain around your neck," is an Ossetian curse which reflects the horror with which the breakup of a family is regarded. In Daghestan, too, the breakup of the family is a common theme in cursing.

MEATS

The place of meat in the Caucasian diet cannot be evaluated without considering its ritual importance in hospitality and feasting. Courtesy demanded that meat be absolutely fresh. The Chechens would kill an animal at the feet of a guest to demonstrate the meat's freshness. "Spilling the blood," as it was called, in a person's honor was a sign of great respect. Just as milk is associated with femininity and motherhood, blood and meat are associated with masculinity. In Abkhasia, when a guest arrives, a woman goes out into the courtyard to catch a chicken to be killed, but if she still menstruates she cannot kill it herself. This must be done by a man.

The animal is carefully dismembered without cutting through bone and roasted on a spit. The head is boiled separately and placed on the table so that guests can see what animal was killed and that the meat is fresh. The

95

head is considered the most honorable part, and half of it goes to the mother's brother, a highly esteemed relative in the Caucasian kinship system. Each piece of meat has its place in a hierarchy of honor, the next most respectable piece being the shoulder and the next, the rib. The heart and liver also have special significance. Toasts to newlyweds are made by the father of the groom and by the oldest relative, holding a ritual stick to which the heart and liver of the sacrificial animal are tied.

Mutton is the most common meat in these sheep-herding cultures. Beef, once scarce and therefore considered more honorable, has become more common with modern improvements in food distribution. Goat meat is also eaten, and pork can be found in non-Moslem areas. Horsemeat was eaten only by some Daghestani groups. Generally, the horse is considered half-human and his blood the same as man's. Georgians and Abkhasians will not touch horsemeat. In battle a horse fights together with his master, trying to pull down the enemy and trample on him with his hooves, or trying to bite him. The idea of a creature half-man and half-horse brings to mind of course the ancient mythology of Greece and other Near Eastern cultures. Fish, despite its abundance in the rivers and in the Caspian Sea, is eaten rarely. It must be remembered that the Caucasians are traditionally a pastoral and agricultural people who retain their ancient habits. Fishing was simply not a part of their heritage and they never developed a taste for fish. Now, however, some efforts are being made to add fish to their diet. To this end, a number of artificial lakes have been built where fish are stocked and bred.

Boiling and roasting are the preferred methods of preparing meat, with frying being most common in Azerbaijan. In remote mountain regions, where animals were driven out to pasture in the summers, the custom of smoking meat in the spring and winter was established. *Shashlyk* or *shishkebab*, a favorite dish of many Caucasians, is roasted over hot coals after the meat has been rubbed with tallow. This method of preparation lets the meat brown rapidly outside while the juices inside are preserved.

BEANS

Since meat was somewhat of a rarity and treat in the past when the standard of living was much lower, high-protein foods such as beans were used widely. Beans continue to be an important component of the diets of all Caucasian peoples. The Chechens eat beans at almost every meal, sometimes with meat. *Lobio* is a popular Abkhasian dish made from red kidney beans, onions, walnuts, and spices. For memorial rituals, a similar dish using lima beans is prepared.

SPICES AND HERBS

Spices and herbs are used extensively everywhere in the Caucasus. Basil, dill, parsley and parsley root, sorrel, peppers, garlic, coriander, mint, and savory are cultivated, with wild-growing plants also being used widely. Some of those plants regarded as weeds in other parts of Europe—purslane, nettles, burdock, horse and sour chives, chabrets, horse beans, dandelions—were gathered by wandering shepherds in the Caucasus, used for food, and later cultivated. Edible grasses are used in salads and as filling for meat pies made from dried meat, cheese, onions, eggs, spices, and vinegar. The concentration of vitamin C in some of these plants ranges from 80 to 190 mg per cent— the daily minimum requirement being in the order of 70 mg per cent*— which gives some idea of the nutritional value of the more than 200 species of edible plants growing wild in the region. Carotene (6.55–11.45 mg per cent) and iron (98–184 mg per cent) are especially plentiful in mint, savory, and coriander. In addition, watercress, dill, leek, coriander, and celery are rich in mineral complexes (19.34–24.73 mg per cent).

In many cultures foraging is felt to be demeaning and something to be done only in the last resort. The Russian curse "You will eat nettles" (meaning that hungry times are coming) illustrates this contempt for foraged foods. The Caucasians, however, consider wild-growing plants such as nettles not only edible, but tasty. As a matter of fact, nettles contain ascorbic acid, carotene, vitamins K and B_{12}, protein and other trace elements. Wild garlic is employed extensively and, as mentioned earlier, prized for its medicinal properties. A Chechen proverb states: "Garlic cures nine diseases." It should be noted that Caucasians use salt sparingly despite their well-developed taste for herbs and spices. In mountain regions, wild-growing herbs rather than spices predominate, while in hot lowland regions, spices are preferred to herbs and marinades.

Dr. L.A. Arutiunian advances an interesting theory as to why the Caucasians use such an abundance of hot spices. At higher climatic temperatures, such as those found in Azerbaijan, for instance, changes in the salt-water- ,

*Many scientists have begun to think the need is often higher, though there is still controversy about what the right amount for each person is.

protein- , fat- , hydrocarbon- , and vitamin-exchange processes occur. There is also a reduction of gastric juices, altering the functions of the digestive tract, the glycogen metabolism in the liver, and the balance of protein in the blood. The appetite is lowered as a result of these disturbances. Stimulating appetite and the secretion of gastric juices with hot spices is a good remedy. The spices contain almost no calories and thus are excellent appetite stimulants, creating the conditions for good digestion.

In Abkhasia, a hot sauce called *adzhika* is prepared from red peppers, salt, dill, garlic, coriander, onions, nuts, damson plums, tomatoes, and beet greens. The mixture is ground on a flat surface with a round stone. It is an aromatic and bitter sauce, reddish-brown in color. Other Caucasian groups prepare similar hot sauces—the Georgian *tkemali* sauce, for instance—which are used sparingly by the old and more generously by the adventurous young. Tart, unripe fruits—damsons among the Abkhasians, sour and cornelian cherries among the Chechens—often flavor these sauces.

Caucasians are very fond of their national sauces and eat them with many different foods. I was once visited in New York by some of my Caucasian colleagues, for whom I prepared an American-style dinner. They enjoyed and praised the meal, but asked whether I didn't have some Caucasian sauces. It so happened that one of these professors had himself given me some *adzhika* when I was in Abkhasia, and I dutifully fetched the vial from the kitchen. The roast chicken was much improved by the *adzhika,* they told me.

NUTS

Nuts are common seasonings. They are grated or crushed for cooking, or eaten whole. Almonds, pecans, walnuts, beech nuts, and hazelnuts—excellent sources of protein, minerals, vitamins, and fats—are cultivated. Chestnuts are collected in great quantities and dried and stored for the winter. In Abkhasia, they are used to make a thick mash which is covered with nut oil and served directly on a clean wooden table. Nut oil is often used instead of butter or animal fat in Abkhasia.

The sauces for beef or mutton are made of ground walnuts, red and black pepper, tart plums, and the juice of unripened grapes. The spices provide the meat with a good aroma and taste. The juice of unripened grapes is very rich in vitamin C and is generally used instead of vinegar. Walnut, highly regarded and used throughout the Caucasus, is also very rich in vitamin C and to a lesser degree in vitamins A and B. The ripened nuts are pressed to extract oil, which is used for cooking. The nuts are 51.9 per cent to 69.9 per cent oil. The protein content is between 14.5 per cent and 24 per cent. Caucasians eat about 30 to 90 grams of walnuts (called Greek nuts in Russian) a day, which completely supplies the fat necessary for human maintenance. Other cultivated and wild nuts provide protein, carbohydrates, vitamins, and minerals.

FRUITS AND VEGETABLES

Fresh fruits and vegetables are cultivated and enjoyed throughout the Caucasus. In the lowland regions, where agriculture flourishes, cultivated fruits and vegetables are most important, while in the mountain regions, children, adults, and especially old people know where wild edible plants can be found. Since freshness is of the utmost concern, people will often simply go out into the garden before breakfast to pick fruit and vegetables for their breakfast salad, complete with onion and garlic. One of my New York colleagues who accompanied me on a trip to the Caucasus at first found this custom of eating morning salads somewhat bizarre. Now she too enjoys morning vegetables.

The favorable climate of the Caucasus makes it a veritable hothouse for tasty and beneficial plants. In Georgia, spinach, lettuce, estragon, celery, sorrel, cucumbers, tomatoes, peppers, eggplant, radishes, beets, potatoes, onions, garlic, watermelons, muskmelons, pumpkins, cabbage, and watercress are cultivated widely. In most areas of the Caucasus grains are also cultivated. Wheat is now the primary grain, but in the past, barley and millet were used to make bread. In Armenia, rice has been grown since ancient times, probably under Persian influence, and pilaf still occupies an important place in the Armenian kitchen.

According to Dr. S.I. Baluev, a Russian gerontologist, ascorbic acid in large doses has the remarkable property of normalizing the level of cholesterol in the blood. Vitamin C may be a factor in the low incidence of arteriosclerosis. People who eat a large amount of fresh vegetables are apparently not nearly as subject to arteriosclerosis as those who do not. "Perhaps," writes Dr. A.L. Miasnikov, "one of the reasons for the longevity of certain peoples in the Caucasus [is that] the large amounts of green vegetables, onion, and garlic which they use are rich sources of vitamin C."

Grape vines grow everywhere in the mountains and the countryside, and the region produces a great deal of wine. Indeed, Abkhasia, together with the rest of Georgia, is known as the vineyard of the U.S.S.R. Every homestead, no matter how poor, has its own vineyard. The popular Isabella grape seems to produce the best wine. During the harvest, which begins in September and may last until January, grapes are such an abundant and favorite food that a man may eat fifty kilograms in a single season. It is said that in autumn, the birds are so happy and stuffed with grapes that they can barely fly. The old people say that the skins and seeds should not be eaten as they are hard to digest, but younger people eat the grapes whole, straight from the vine. Grapes are included in many popular main dishes.

HONEY AND SWEETS

Honey, as I've said before, is used widely in Caucasian folk medicine and more recently has been adopted for therapeutic use by the Soviet medical profession. Nutritionally, it is an excellent source of sugars, notably wine sugar. In addition to being highly caloric, honey is said to contain more than twelve different vitamins as well as hormones, microelements, and mineral salts. It also possesses bactericidal and antibiotic properties and facilitates detoxification of microorganisms. Honey is added to milk, sour milk, tea, mineral water, and is also used in cooking.

Candy and sweets are not common in the Caucasus, since granulated sugar is something of a novelty there. The Chechens, however, prepare a kind of *halva* which has been eaten since ancient times. Roasted-wheat flour is mixed with honey and hot oil and placed in a warm spot. When the candy is cool, it is rolled out into a block and cut into pieces. Because of the premium placed on freshness, the preservation of fruit in sugar—jams, jellies, and so forth— is uncommon.

TEETH

Most Caucasians—especially in rural areas—have strong teeth and keep them for most of their lives. This may be due to the absence of refined sugar in their diet and to the large amounts of roughage, which requires a lot of chewing.

MILK PRODUCTS AND SPRING WATER

Matzoni, a yogurt-like cultured milk, is considered an aid to digestion generally and a remedy for stomach disorders. Caucasians take *matzoni* after virtually every meal, especially if they think the food is difficult to digest. *Matzoni* is prepared from either cow, goat, sheep, or buffalo milk, both fresh and boiled. Unlike other milk cultures, it has a curd which breaks down readily into extremely small particles that are easily digested. Therefore, it is an ideal food for the very young and very old and for those with digestive problems. *Matzoni* grains, resembling small, spongy grains of rice, and starter consisting of milk solids and microorganisms (bacillus caucasicum and streptococcus A, in particular) are used for starting the fermentation. A few spoonfuls from a previous batch of *matzoni* or fresh cottage cheese without preservatives may also be used as a starter. Sometimes the cheeselike formation found in the stomach of a young calf that has eaten nothing but its mother's milk is dried and made into a starter.

In western Georgia, the most prosperous section of the republic and the section with the highest incidence of longevity, over two pounds of cheese and other milk products are consumed daily per capita. The Chechens eat a large amount of lightly salted cottage cheese. In the cities and towns of Armenia, cheese is eaten virtually every day, sometimes several times a day. Pieces of cheese are wrapped in *lavash,* similar to Syrian bread, or eaten with fruits as a snack or as dessert—to "gild the mouth," as the old people say. In the past in Armenia, bread and cheese were a staple. In Daghestan, large amounts of cheese and farmer's cheese are eaten. In the mountains, cheeses are made from both goat and sheep milk and kept in burlap, or molded into large discs and wrapped in special grass and hay.

Airan (sour milk diluted with water) and sour cream are other common cultured milk products.

There are firm rules as to when fresh milk should be drunk. The Abkhasians believe that fish and fresh milk together are poisonous, and the classical Azerbaijanian poet, Nizami Tiandzhevi, writes in his work, *Iskender Name:*

When you are having vinegar, don't drink milk;
Milk and vinegar aren't good for you.

Spring water is also universally prized in the Caucasus. Villages are usually near a spring, but if not, the Caucasians go out of their way to get spring water. It is especially extolled by the old people.

FOOD PREPARATION AND PRESERVATION

The methods of meat-cooking favored in the Caucasus, roasting and boiling, tend to eliminate excess fat. In roasting, the fat drips into the fire and in boiling, continued until the blood ceases to flow, most of the fat is rendered from the meat. The Abkhasians consider the broth which remains after boiling unhealthy, but some Caucasian groups use the broth for soups. Chicken is cooked only until the meat turns white and the blood ceases to flow. Smoking was used in Daghestan and other mountainous areas to preserve meats, since the flocks were out in distant summer pastures for most of the year. In other areas, smoked meat was used primarily on military expeditions. Where frying is common, chiefly in Azerbaijan, animal fats rather than the vegetable oils are used. Lamb or mutton fat is employed, but the less digestible beef fat is avoided. Pork fat is forbidden in the Moslem dietary laws. Lamb fat is used much as we use butter and margarine. When vegetables are served with meat, for example, a small dent is made in the vegetables to hold the fat.

In cooking, fastidious cleanliness is the rule everywhere. Although some groups still eat with their fingers, ritual washing before meals is often practiced.

The continued use of wooden utensils, despite the influx of modern metal kitchen utensils, is also noteworthy. Wood is preferred, as it does not impart a metallic taste to the food.

Vegetables and fruits are not sliced but eaten whole whenever possible. Nutritional experts have told me that shredding or grating causes vitamin C to oxidize rapidly. Old Caucasians simply say whole fruits and raw or only slightly cooked vegetables taste better.

TEA

The use of tea came north from Iran into Azerbaijan, and from there spread throughout the Caucasus. Tea is grown in many areas of the Caucasus but, except in Moslem areas, it is rarely used by the indigenous population, who are usually devoted to the local wine. In some areas, tea has a ritualistic importance parallel to that of wine for toasting. Among the Chechens tea with milk—*Kalmyk* tea—is drunk regularly at breakfast. If one does not have his own tea, he goes to the home of a neighbor or relative to drink tea in the morning. Azerbaijanian doctors make the same claims for the beneficial action of tea as other Caucasian doctors make for wine. According to Dr. M. Sultanov, for example, the opinion that the caffeine in strong tea harms the heart is unfounded. It has been shown, he says, that tea has a tonic effect on the heart and is actually even more beneficial than caffeine injections for the treatment of strokes, hypertension, and arteriosclerosis. Tea also normalizes sleep patterns. According to Dr. Sultanov:

Caffeine gives tea its thirst-quenching properties, eliminates the feeling of tiredness, improves the disposition, and facilitates digestion. Vitamin R, especially abundant in tea, rectifies capillary toxicosis, capillary breakage, low permeability of vessel walls, and arteriosclerosis. It is impossible to imagine supper or breakfast, not to mention festive occasions, without velvety, aromatic tea.

Tea contains a whole number of valuable substances—tannic acid (a bactericide), thiamine, nicotinic acid, vitamins B_1, B_2, C, and R, and tea ash which contains many vital trace elements, including potassium and phosphorus. The maximal amounts, however, are available only in properly brewed tea. Tea brewed directly in boiling water contains only the coloring and flavoring substances, according to Dr. Sultanov. He recommends the following Azerbaijanian recipe for tea: A small teapot for essence is rinsed out twice with boiling water and one teaspoon of tea per adult placed in the pot, which is now one-third filled with cool boiled water and placed on top of a large pot of boiling water, as in a Russian samovar. The large pot is allowed to boil for twenty minutes, and the essence pot is then removed, covered with a thick cloth, and allowed to stand for an additional five minutes. The essence is diluted in the cup with some of the hot water. The tea is drunk strong and in great quantity; Sultanov recommends two cups in the morning, one at noon, and one with the evening meal.

CHANGES IN NUTRITION AND DIET DURING THE SOVIET PERIOD

In the past, diet varied tremendously from one type of economy to another. The nomadic pastoral diet consisted primarily of different varieties of meats and foraged fruits and vegetables. Starchy foods were not significant; some nomads were even unwilling to eat bread. But the agricultural people of the plains ate cultivated vegetables and grains. Hippocrates reported that the people of the Caucasus lived on cherries, pine cones, apples, melons, and berries which grew wild in the woods. Even at that time the area was famous for longevity, and the Greeks may have sought dietary clues to why these peoples attained such unusual ages.

It is yet to be seen whether the changes that have occurred in the diets of the Caucasian peoples since the Revolution will affect the incidence of longevity. It is believed that the dietary patterns established early and maintained throughout life have an overwhelming significance in longevity. An analysis of the diet of seventy-eight men and forty-five women aged one hundred and over showed little dietary change in their lifetimes. They had consumed mostly milk and vegetables (74 per cent of intake) and protein in moderation. The total absence of idiosyncratic food preferences among the long-living demonstrates first, the complete coincidence of cultural options and individual preferences, and, second, the premium placed on discipline and self-control in Caucasian cultures. It is interesting that the longevous, who eat the same kinds of food their entire lives—the same foods which their ancestors at the time of Hippocrates were eating—enjoy and prefer it. This coincidence of option and preference, however, develops only because of the emphasis placed on discipline in all aspects of life. In a society such as the Chechen, for instance, where a child will give up a favorite dish for a week simply to test his self-discipline, finicky eaters who have to be coaxed with new foods are not likely to develop.

Nowadays, the widespread distribution of products in a complex economy, the introduction of vegetable cultivation in the mountainous areas, and especially the rural trading network have made different kinds of foods available throughout the Caucasus. Diets have become more uniform year-round and less dependent on seasonal crops. Macaroni, sugar (instead of honey), and manufactured pastries which were unknown in the past have come into common use. Special dishes for children are served today, in keeping with modern medical thought. In the past, infants and young children were fed the same food as the rest of the family. Now parents, instructed by doctors, give their children milk, eggs, and other vitamin-rich foods. But despite these changes, the traditional national dishes remain the favorites, and the old dietary customs are for the most part still preserved.

MEDICAL REPORTS: CORONARY INSUFFICIENCY, ARTERIOSCLEROSIS, CHOLESTEROL

Soviet gerontologists and physicians are studying food patterns to establish correlations between diseases of the circulatory system and diet. In the Soviet Union, as in other industrialized countries, the mortality due to these diseases is on the rise. Arteriosclerosis in conjunction with hypertension is considered one of the greatest causes of pathological aging.

Dr. I.N. Daraseliya studied the relationship between diet and coronary insufficiency among Abkhasian industrial and agricultural workers. The study group included 522 men between the ages of forty and fifty-nine, among whom ten showed coronary insufficiency. Eight of these were industrial workers and two were collective farmers. Between the ages of forty and forty-nine, three industrial workers showed coronary insufficiency; between fifty and fifty-nine, five industrial workers and two collective farmers showed coronary insufficiency. The median level of blood cholesterol was higher in the industrial workers. On the average, the industrial workers consumed 24 per cent more food, but only half as much vitamin C as the agricultural workers.

The highest frequency of arteriosclerosis, in the opinion of many investigators, is observed among persons who eat large quantities of animal fat. Animal fats are heavy in cholesterol. Vegetable fats often lower the level of hypercholesterolemia and help prevent the development of arteriosclerosis.

Research on the role of alimentary fats and cholesterol in the pathogenesis of arteriosclerosis among elderly persons, as well as among longevous persons, was carried out by Dr. M.N. Sultanov. Dr. Sultanov conducted clinical examinations of over 300 Azerbaijanians, divided into sex, age, and occupational categories. These subjects had similar life-styles and diet. The average amount of animal fat consumed was approximately 125 ± 8.9 grams per day. They ate no vegetable fat at all.

The study of cholesterol-protein-hydrocarbon exchange involved 154 persons, forty-three of whom were "advanced adult," thirty-five of whom were "old," and seventy-six of whom were "long-living." The control group was people twenty-five to fifty-nine years old.

Low cholesterol levels were found in all of the age groups, with the norm of 150–180 mg per cent as compared with the American male norm of 240 mg per cent. Among people twenty-five to thirty-nine years old the average level of cholesterol was 97.1 ± 9.3 mg per cent. In the older age groups there was a noteworthy increase. For persons fifty to fifty-nine years the level was 115.7 ± 3.6 mg per cent. In the advanced-adult and old-age groups there was a marked trend toward a lower cholesterol level, and among long-living people the level was 91.8 ± 4.2 mg per cent.

It has been established that increased cholesterol in the diet suppresses excessive cholesterol synthesis within the body. Sultanov believes that animal fats stimulate the breakdown of fat, and strengthen the regulatory mechanisms of exchange, thus inhibiting the synthesis of endogenous cholesterol.

In Azerbaijan, famous for longevity, a high-cholesterol diet is traditional. The Nagorny-Karabakh, and Nakhichevan A.S.S.R. (mountainous areas) deserve special mention. The low incidence (4.8 per cent) of arteriosclerosis with related hypertension in Nakhichevan A.S.S.R., where for each 100,000 population there are 592 longevous people (1967), supports Sultanov's results.

According to Sultanov, arteriosclerosis cannot be the result of a high-cholesterol diet. But the interrelationships between the amount of cholesterol in the diet, the amount the body itself produces, and the level of cholesterol in the blood are at best poorly understood. There is clearly not a one-to-one relationship between the amount of cholesterol taken into the body and the cholesterol levels in the blood. Even so, most scientists accept the idea that excessive dietary cholesterol, while it may decrease the body's own production to some extent, nevertheless usually results in an excess in the blood and the eventual clogging of blood vessels.

A recent nutritional study of the Masai tribesmen of East Africa yielded surprising results suggesting that yogurt may reduce cholesterol in the blood, although yogurt, like whole milk, is a high-cholesterol food, a quart containing 120 to 150 mg. The Masai are unusually resistant to heart disease and have very low blood-cholesterol levels, averaging 135 mg per cent (as against the American male average of 240 mg per cent) despite a heavy milk and meat diet.

During the study the Masai, who normally consume a quart of yogurt a day, were given twice that amount, and in some cases more. The blood-cholesterol levels dropped significantly during the study. In fact, the more yogurt consumed, the greater was the drop, despite the tremendous increase in dietary cholesterol. This cholesterol-lowering effect has since been reproduced in adult Americans who are being fed large amounts of home-made yogurt. It is believed that the yogurt bacteria produce a substance, probably a fatty acid, that blocks cholesterol production in the liver, although this substance has not yet been isolated.

The research team was quick to emphasize that diet is certainly not the only factor that protects the Masai from heart disease. For instance, the average Masai walks up to twenty-five miles a day, and even the very old walk eight to ten miles.

The study of the Masai is useful in our search for the causes of Caucasian longevity because of the similarities in two important elements, diet and exercise. Both groups, in general, consume large quantities of a yogurt-like milk culture, and both walk great distances in the course of their daily lives. No simplistic conclusions can be drawn, but these striking parallels cannot be ignored.

I found that nutrition in Caucasia varied considerably, not only from one ethnic group to the next, but often even within the same ethnic group in different regions. Dr. G.Z. Pitskhelauri spent many hours with me explaining the basic differences between food patterns in western and eastern Georgia, in terms of caloric intake and chemical and vitamin composition. The extreme longevity and good health enjoyed in western Georgia is in marked contrast to the lower longevity and somewhat less robust health recorded in eastern Georgia.

D.F. Dzhorbenadze and M.I. Zurabashvili, both of the Research Institute of Physiology and Pathology of Women in Tbilisi, studied the differences in diet between the eastern and western zones of Georgia during summer and fall.

Khatyndzhan-nana, a 128-year-old man of the village Sheikhmakhmud, told Professor Sultanov:

All the members of our family love meat and milk dishes. A glass of *matzoni* before going to bed helps put you to sleep and is good for your stomach. Our tasty peas are also very nutritious. As soon as someone recovers from an illness we begin to feed him peas; after a couple of days, he is completely well—right before your very eyes. Believe me, our food improves our health in many different ways, especially the dishes made from peas. Because of this, if you ever need to improve your health quickly, eat peas. Herbs and marinates improve our appetite. In our house we eat moderately with good appetite. As one Azerbaijanian saying says: "If you want respect, don't talk too much; if you want health, don't eat too much." Gluttony, like laziness, is man's enemy.

TABLE 10: Dietary Differences Between East and West Georgia

Eastern Zone	Western Zone
Wheat products, 410 g/day	Wheat products, 217 g/day
Potatoes, 143 g/day	Potatoes 98, g/day
Vegetable and fruit products used extensively in both zones.	
Meat (2 times more than in Western Zone)	No soups
Large quantity of animal fats.	Meat, broiled
Beef fat used. Generally, the	Ground nuts used as spices
amount of animal fat used in the	replacing use of fat.
Eastern Zone is 1.3 times more	
than that used in the West.	
Milk products, 272 g	Milk products, 517.6 g
Cheese, 32 g	Cheese, 65.6 g
Sugar, 13.5 g	Sugar, 7.8 g
	Honey, 11.4 g
Total calories, 1777	Total calories, 1947
Total protein, 72 g	Total protein, 84 g

In another interesting study done by M.N. Sultanov, D.G. Tagdisi, B.K. Shakuri, and A.V. Ragimov, it was learned that there is a certain interdependence between the concentration of trace elements and the number of people of "advanced adult," "old," and "long-living" groups in some areas of Nakhichevan. It has been established that either a deficiency or an excess of certain trace elements encourages disorders of various physiological functions with the resultant development of diseases. Vitamins are activated by certain trace elements—zinc, manganese, copper, cobalt, and molybdenum, most importantly. These trace elements are present in the soil, vegetation, and water in differing amounts in the various regions. They are of unknown importance in longevity.

Research done by Drs. Chebotarev and Sachuk elucidates the interrelationship between diseases and their aftereffects in old age. Infectious diseases (scarlet fever, diphtheria, typhus, malaria, chicken pox, and so forth) leave definite traces in the organism even into old age and affect health. Poor general health and a high susceptibility to diseases of the heart, and circulatory and respiratory system were found in the group which had experienced early illnesses. Thus, the cumulative effect of serious illness can be seen as one of the factors affecting longevity.

EXERCISE

Dr. Sultanov suggests that the performance of the *namaz*, ritual prayer (required five times a day from the age of ten), in addition to its religious significance is a strenuous physical exercise which may contribute to the physical well-being and longevity of the Moslem Azerbaijanians.

The prayer is preceded by the ceremonial washing of the face, the hands, and the feet with water, or with sand if no water is available, according to a set form. The worshippers always face Mecca. The prayer begins with a standing position, the hands beside the head with fingers extended. The next postures are a half-seated, half-kneeling position and prostration with the toes and knees on the ground, the hands extended flat beside the head and the forehead usually touching a small "prayer stone," often made of baked earth from some holy place. The half-seated, half-kneeling position is resumed for the conclusion of the prayer, which may be said in any clean place but is often recited on a mat or rug intended for the purpose.

The exact hours at which the *namaz* is said vary in different parts of the Muslim world, but it is always preceded by the call to prayer by the *muezzin* from the mosque or minaret. Recently a loudspeaker has been used in some countries to broadcast the call to prayer. The times are: dawn, before sunrise; noon, just after the sun has passed the zenith; afternoon, before sunset—often midafternoon; at sunset; and after dark.

In the ancient past, the prayers of the Moslems were developed not only for religious purposes but with an eye to the development of powerful warriors with good endurance. This may explain the "gymnastic" aspect of the Islamic prayers.

7
SEX: JOY IN PRIVATE, SHAME IN PUBLIC

It is very difficult to gather specific sexual data from Caucasians, and quite naturally so. Their reticence to reveal personal sexual matters cannot be separated from their very strong aversion to overt expressions of emotion and to all public display of physical affection between family members, and especially between married couples. There are strict rules of avoidance between husband and wife in the presence of others, especially old relatives. In the past, even the public acknowledgment of parenthood was avoided. I myself was never asked whether I was married, divorced, or widowed. I had to volunteer answers without having been directly questioned.

The modesty associated with sex is carried over into labor and childbirth. The husband, now as in the past, leaves the house at the onset of labor, avoiding even taking his wife to the hospital, and does not return home until she has completely recovered. In Abkhasia, a husband will take his wife to the hospital if she breaks her arm, but never if she is to give birth. During labor and childbirth, the husband, as the folk expression goes, "gets shy."

Just as almost every aspect of their lives is formalized and supported by ritual and etiquette, so is sex. It is felt that exposing sexual feelings to public view destroys its special quality—like "stripping a flower of its petals and leaving it naked," as one Chechen friend expressed it to me. Desire, they say, should be locked in your heart.

Men and women do not gossip casually about their sexual relations. A woman would never brag about her husband's sexual prowess, nor would a man joke with his cronies about his sex life.

The Caucasian concern with propriety and correct behavior made it difficult for people to discuss sexual matters with me. For example, in Abkhasia, my associate, an anthropologist quite a bit younger than I, could not bring

111

himself to tell me that my sleeveless dress would be considered highly indecent in the villages since the Abkhasians regard the armpit as an erogenous
zone. Exposing one's underarms, I later learned, is almost as improper as
uncovering one's breast.

The difficulty of investigating sexual patterns in the Caucasus was still
further complicated by the rather puritanical Soviet attitudes toward sex.
Thus, although I had read and heard that bestiality was prevalent in the
Caucasus because of late marriage and the importance attached to women's
virginity, it was difficult to initiate a conversation on this theme with any of
my Soviet colleagues.

An Abkhasian friend, late for an appointment with me, explained that he
had just come from a funeral. "You know," he said, "the son-in-law of the
she-goat." I knew that the man to whom he referred was a bachelor in his
forties who lived alone. It was known in the village that he kept a she-goat
and her young offspring for the purpose of sodomy. The sharp-tongued
villagers had, therefore, assigned him his nickname.

Although sex is considered a good, pleasurable, and guiltless matter when
it is strictly private, there is a feeling of uneasiness, shame, and even danger
connected with any manifestation of sex in the presence of others. This is as
true for the married as the unmarried. When a wife is in a room with her
husband, for example, they keep their voices low so that no one will be able
to hear that they are together.

Privacy and modesty are primary values in the upbringing of children.
Parents never share a bed with older children and, if possible, each child is
given a separate room. Likewise, there is a separate private hut in Abkhasia
—the *amhara* or "silent house"—where newlyweds live.

Although, as we shall see, there are certain absolute standards and rules
in courtship—even an accidental touch by a boy is enough to offend a girl's
family, for example—the discipline is not imposed from outside, but stems
from a respect for privacy and individuality. Thus, a man would consider
himself uncontrolled if he were to take a woman's hand, and the woman
would feel insulted. Since correct behavior continues even in private, restraint
is clearly not merely a matter of social compulsion.

People unfamiliar with the rigid separation of the sexes in the Caucasus
may wonder why in dancing, for instance, even lightly touching a woman was
considered offensive to her family and an insult to herself. (And in rural areas
this is still so.) The teen-age games and routines which we are so accustomed
to, and which prepare young people by more or less gradual means for mature
sexual life, do not exist there, not even in the cities. There is no dating and

necking or touching, or dancing in close embrace at all. So when they do touch, it is a very intense experience which releases pent-up emotions and profound sexual desires.

A Chechen man may promise to wait a whole year or longer after the wedding before exercising his sexual rights. If he approaches his wife ahead of time, she may taunt him with "You promised not to touch me for a year, but you didn't have the strength of will!" In many Caucasian groups sex life and frequency of intercourse are often determined by the woman. If the man should make sexual advances without permission, the wife is very offended. It is considered bad manners for a husband to force himself on his wife without having first received some signal of consent or invitation from her. Even today, the Caucasians believe that discipline and self-denial in sex, especially for men, makes for greater sexual gratification. Thus, the patriarchal life-style does not mean sexual domination by the male.

The internalization of sexual norms is reinforced by a system of formal standards to which all are expected to adhere, regardless of inclination. Dancing, for example, is highly ritualized and regulated. The man circles his partner without touching her, his hands pointed away from her. Even brushing against her scarf would be insulting to her family. Since generally only unmarried women dance, dancing is an integral part of courtship. Among the Cherkessians, the partners separate slowly, facing each other, and return to their places with small dignified steps.

Highly formalized avoidance patterns are another aspect of Caucasian sexuality. It is indecent for a daughter-in-law to address, or look directly at, her father-in-law, and vice-versa. These patterns vary in stringency and extent in different groups, but among all peoples overt manifestations of affection between husband and wife in the presence of other people is absolutely forbidden.

In Abkhasia, after the marriage is consummated, the groom goes to his father and offers him a glass of wine. If the father accepts, the groom is permitted to join the family at dinner. He also gives presents to his relatives. These gifts are called "ransom," and are supposed to cover his shame. It is still considered polite for a groom to stay out of the sight of his older relatives on his wedding night.

In the regions of Northern Caucasus (Kabarda, Balkaria, and others) after it becomes known that the marriage has been consummated, the groom's family invites the most respected elderly relatives and neighbors to its house. The groom and his friends must wait at the door until the elders are seated. The oldest among them opens the door and welcomes the groom, saying that they forgive him his deed and accept his bride. As a sign of forgiveness, the groom receives a large glass of wine and a plate of goodies. He drinks the wine and passes the plate to his companions.

Among the Kabardinians, a town crier announces to the people of the village that the groom wishes to "ransom" himself. Young and old gather in the square, where the bridegroom provides drink and food to be enjoyed by all: wine, several rams roasting on a spit, and fruits of the season.

Virginity before marriage is an absolute necessity for a Caucasian woman. Loss of virginity ends her hope of marriage (except to a less desirable man many years later) and can lead to bloody vendettas against her despoiler. Among the Chechens, if a man touches a woman, she is considered his wife. In Azerbaijan, seeing a woman's eyebrows was considered tantamount to marriage; hence the custom of veiling the face. Among many peoples, a physical relationship was recognized as a common-law marriage; the actual wedding could come later. Among others, the relatives of a couple having premarital sexual relations would try to shame them and force a marriage. Only if a man mistreated and abandoned a woman would there be bloody reprisals.

Caucasians are extremely legal-minded and are well-versed in the laws relating to sexual practices. Today several overlapping codes of law exist. The *adats* or customary law is used throughout the area. A person who transgresses the *adats* is exiled from the community with the understanding that the injured party and his closest relatives have the right to receive a legally specified payment, to kill the accused, or to forgive. Sexual practices are covered under the traditional *adats*. The more serious the crime, the greater the number of relatives required to participate. Orthodox Moslems obey the religious law of the Koran in addition to the *adats*. And, of course, modern Soviet laws apply in the Caucasus. The Soviet authorities, however, do not interfere with the traditional laws except in cases of major crimes such as assault, rape, and murder.

For example, sexual relations not sanctioned by marriage are contrary to the *adats*. If a man returns home and finds another man having sexual relations with his wife, daughter, sister, or mother, he may immediately kill both guilty parties. Laws against adultery are harsh and cruel, because of concern for the purity of the family line and inheritance in it. Also, the honor of the husband is at stake.

In some areas, a husband who commits adultery is also punished, although less severely. He might be fined or his wife might leave him.

Men do not prove their masculinity by collecting women, but they may stray occasionally. It is a point of pride, however, for women never to show jealousy. Extramarital affairs are not permissible for women since the honor of the house is seen to rest with the wife. As long as she is honorable, her husband feels that his honor and pride are safe, no matter what he himself does. A woman who knows of her husband's affairs but maintains a proud silence is much esteemed by her husband and the community.

If an engaged woman runs away with another man of her own free will, she may be brought back by her relatives. Her fiancé may still want to marry her. If she refuses to marry him, her parents must repay twice the bride price. Her lover is not responsible to her fiancé or to her relatives, but the local village elders may levy a fine of two bulls. If the woman is pregnant from this man, he must marry her and give his name to the child. If there is only a suspicion that he has had relations with her, forty of his relatives must join him in the oath to clear his name. I asked Dr. Gardanov, an Ossetian, what would happen if a man's relatives decided not to swear to his innocence or not to leave a village with him. Dr. Gardanov was speechless at such a naive question. Then he said, "Nobody asks a relative. He simply has to. Just as any other relative would have to do it for him."

The *adats* requires the virginity of a bride. If a husband claims that his bride was not a virgin on the wedding night, it must first be established whether he was drunk or sober at the time. If it can be confirmed by those present at the wedding that he was drunk, then the court denies his claim on grounds that establishing virginity is a rather delicate procedure and an intoxicated man may not be able to judge correctly. If the husband does not wish to remain with the bride, he must pay back the dowry money, compensate for all the money spent on the wedding, and return all goods allowed by the marriage contract. But if witnesses testify that the man was sober, his sworn word is accepted. In this case, he has the right to send his bride back to her parents and returns her dowry.

If it is established that during the betrothal period the couple met secretly, any later claim that she was not a virgin is rejected. However, if it can be proven that during the engagement, the woman met with another man and it was noticed that she displayed a certain liking for him, then the husband's accusation is taken seriously.

For a long time, I suspected that there must be some homosexuality in areas where women were strictly secluded, and where it was very difficult to come close to a woman sexually—or even socially. When I examined the published *adats,* I found the punishments for homosexual rape and other sexual abuses spelled out in great detail.

115

In Daghestan the following sexual code was in force until the time of the Soviets:

1. If a man is accused of having sexual relations with an unmarried woman, he must appear, with relatives, before a council of the elders of the community. The relatives must swear to his innocence or admit his guilt. If he is found guilty, he and the woman must each pay a fine of one bull to the community chest.

2. If a man has relations with another man's wife, the punishment is much more severe. In addition to paying a fine to the community chest, both are subject to prosecution by the injured husband and his relatives. The punishment may be the death of the guilty parties. The husband chooses the punishment. He may cut off his wife's nose or he may be merciful and cut off only the sleeves of her dress to shame her in front of the community. At any rate, she can not stay with him any longer. She can go to live with her own family—if they will have her.

3. Homosexuality is punished only when it is practiced in the form of rape; otherwise, it is simply ignored. If a man is accused of forcing sexual relations on a small boy, the law requires that seven relatives swear to his innocence. But if the accusers request it, twelve relatives may be necessary. The family of the boy has a right to kill the man if he is found guilty. This punishment also applies in the rape of a grown man or woman. However, in these cases, witnesses are required.

4. If a man plans to rape a woman, or even if he only touches her, the offense is as punishable as an actual rape.

5. If a man over fifteen years of age is accused of bestiality, witnesses are required to prove his innocence or guilt. If there are no witnesses, six relatives may swear to his innocence. A man found guilty must pay a money fine and must give the owner another animal of the same kind. For boys under fifteen, bestiality is not considered an offense.

It is interesting to note the part played by relatives in protecting and helping the accused. In many cases, relatives are held responsible as a group. In blood feuds, the avengers may kill any relative of the accused if they cannot find the guilty individual.

The modern Abkhasian novel *Sandro of Georgia* by Fazil Iskander, is the story of a young Abkhasian couple who elope against the wishes of their parents. They manage to slip away during a feast and when the news reaches the collective farm where the feast is taking place, the young men are especially furious. They snatch up their weapons and leap onto their horses. When they reach the edge of the village, following the only trail along which the lovers could have gone, the village elder orders the men to halt. He dismounts and walks a few steps down the trail to a small grove where he sees a patch of matted grass. He returns to his men. "They have already succeeded," he tells them. A young man says, "They should have been ashamed to make love in front of the horses." "What for? They are now husband and wife—why should they be ashamed?" the old man replies. The young men return, disappointed, to the village.

This story demonstrates that although abduction is a common reason for spilling blood, the Caucasians generally respect or make allowances for human feelings by legitimizing an accomplished action. The story is also interesting in the way it portrays the different age groups. Playing their expected roles, the young men are hot-headed and ready for action while the old man calms them down. Actually, marriage by capture was familiar among the Caucasians, for two main reasons: first, the bride price may be too high for the young man to pay and second, capturing a bride is considered manly and courageous.

Areas under the greatest influence from Islam, with its oppression of women, impose the greatest sexual restrictions on women. In Azerbaijan, the most orthodox of the Moslem areas, where the Shiite sect had great influence, a woman was killed by her brother for an extra- or premarital affair. Restrictions on bright-colored clothing, dancing, uncovered heads, and appearing on the street without veils were even stricter than in other areas of the Caucasus. In other Moslem areas, however, a woman was rarely punished by death for her sexual behavior except for incest, an unforgivable sin among all Caucasian groups.

SEX AND LONGEVITY

In old age, self-discipline and moderation continue to be the values which regulate sexual life. The Caucasians expect to live long, healthy, and creative lives; self-discipline is necessary to conserve their energies. Since abstinence is believed to prolong sexual potency, regular sexual relations are expected to start late in life. Postponement of satisfaction is not deemed frustrating, but rather a promise of future enjoyment. Sexual activity continuing into old age is as natural as a healthy appetite or sound sleep. Celibacy is regarded to a certain extent as abnormal, antisocial, and contrary to human nature— and in fact very few of the long-living are unmarried.

The pattern of late marriage, with the husband usually considerably older than his wife, is changing in the Caucasus. More and more people are marrying in their twenties instead of waiting to the more "proper" age of thirty. (It should be noted that along with falling birth rates and marriage ages has come a drop in the number of longevous people over the past twenty years.) However, the Caucasians do appear to be physiologically "late bloomers." To Westerners, young Caucasian people often seem much younger than they actually are.

Great age differences between husband and wife are not strange in the least. Chechen men sometimes marry women fifty or sixty years younger than themselves. Magomed Khosiev, a Chechen ethnographer, told me of a case of a 120-year-old man marrying a forty-year-old woman and fathering three children.

Many longevous people retain their reproductive function. Ali-Kishi, of the village Kirpi in the Dzhulpinski region of Nakhichevan, at the age of seventy-nine, married a young woman who bore him five children, the last when he was ninety-six. A medical team investigating the sex life of the Abkhasians found that many men retain their sexual potency far beyond the age of seventy. Also, 13.6 per cent of the women continued menstruation after age fifty-five. Late menarche and menopause both indicate a slow aging process.

Although no stigma is attached to a young woman's having an elderly husband, few women are married to much younger men. Obviously, the motivation for a marriage between an older woman and a young man would be purely romantic. Throughout the Caucasus, I heard it said repeatedly that if there are desire and strength, age is never a barrier to sexuality.

Gerontologist R.A. Alikishiev, interested in the sex life of longevous people, reports that Hadju Murtazaliev, a Daghestanian, married for the third time when he was ninety. He had thirteen children by this marriage, and his wife is very pleased with her family life. When questioned, she praised her husband's unusually good disposition.

When Alikishiev asked about the intensity of marital relations for the long-living people, they all reported that a proper restraint is necessary. They feel that one should not stop having marital relations, regardless of chronological age, because one does not stop being a man or woman at any given time. They also feel that if one stops for any length of time, it is much harder to resume sexual activity in late life.

The median age for the long-living people in Daghestan, according to

Alikishiev, is 81.9 for a man. Out of seventy-nine people interviewed, seventeen had potency up to 100 to 127 years of age. Budichi Ramazanov, aged 135, from the village of Vatchi, testified that his sex life ceased when he was 127. Alikishiev gives a long list of very old people who state that they are potent and have a normal sex life.

8
THE FAMILY:
THE EXTENDED
FAMILY OF THE PAST,
THE SMALL UNITS
OF TODAY

For Caucasians, the most intense and involved relationship both now and in the past is that of an individual with his family. One's very existence is inextricably woven into the fabric of an interdependent, mutually supportive group of relatives, extended family, and community. There is no identity for an individual outside of this intricate network. The importance of belonging to the family, and through the family to the lineage, cannot be exaggerated. The idea of escaping from the family or striking out on one's own was alien, probably because rebellion was difficult and generally futile. There are few, if any, alternatives to the communal life of the family. A rare man might become a mountain outlaw or a war hero but few aspired to the loneliness that awaited one outside the community. For a woman, there were no options. Exclusion from the family remains the gravest punishment. One never ceases to belong except for some unpardonable crime such as incest or disloyalty to the family, in which case the family name is taken away, a fate considered tantamount to death.

The tradition of family loyalty holds firm despite the inroads of modern industrialization and Soviet law. Even though now there are opportunities for training and jobs, it is still economically and emotionally advantageous to belong to the family. In the Caucasus, the family, whether the traditional, multigenerational extended family or the more modern nuclear family, is still a powerful institution, offering comfort and security from cradle to grave.

The extended families which characterized Caucasian society in the past were well-organized, structured territorial communities. The extended family was the basic social unit, unified by a common name, and committed to mutual aid, economic support and cooperation, participation in blood feuds, revenge, hospitality, and the family cult. The extended family was patrilineal and, with rare exceptions, patrilocal. Among the Ossetians, a propertyless groom might move into the house of the bride's parents and work off the bride price (the *kalym*) for several years. But usually the sons' brides came to live in the father's house. Not only the name, but also the inheritance with all its traditional complexities passed through the father's line. A family of four or five generations numbering fifty or more people might all live together. These families were of two general patrilineal types: an old man, his sons, their wives and children, and his unmarried daughters; or an old man and his brothers and their patrilineal descendants, their sons and unmarried daughters. An Armenian characterized the extended family as "a little state." Five-, six-, and even seven-generation communes were preserved in the highlands, where the peasant family lived in isolation with its natural economy and where the patriarchal way of life was retained until the late nineteenth century. In modified form the extended family continues today because it offers two principal advantages: economic security and physical and emotional safety.

In the extended family, regardless of size, all of the married couples lived together. Among some nationalities they lived in various rooms of a single house; among others they lived in separate buildings clustered around a single courtyard. Work was under the direction of the oldest man and woman, the man leading the male group and the woman the female group. The division of labor among the sexes had its peculiarities in different regions but basically the men took care of agriculture and animal husbandry while the women had charge of housework as well as certain cottage industries. Children and adolescents helped the adults.

The pastoral and agricultural basis of mountain society required a large group capable of dividing the various tasks involved in wine-growing, animal husbandry, domestic chores, agriculture, and so on. Many hands with diverse talents were needed for survival. Specializations within the family developed. Some women, for instance, might be skilled at weaving, others at sewing, weapon-making, cooking, leather-making, and so on. Shepherds took animals to distant mountain pastures during the summer months and remained there with them. The land had to be plowed, planted, and harvested.

The extended family also functioned as a military unit, defending itself or uniting with other families against common enemies. The pressures of constant warfare and poverty made it absolutely essential that there be no conflict within the lineage.

The lack of centralized authority throughout most of its history strengthened the extended family in the Caucasus. The weaker the overall centralized system, the larger and stronger the family lineage.

When an extended family grew too large, sons or grandsons often settled next to the old compound. Even today, there are many whole villages inhabited by people related to one another and conscious of their common origin and kinship. Recently, with the rise of the nuclear family and the industrialization of many areas, young couples have begun to settle separately and establish their own households, but the traditional obligations and prerogatives linking each individual with the family are still taken seriously.

In other peasant cultures, sons sometimes come into conflict with the father because they wish to be independent of his authority or because they want to receive their share of land sooner than the father is willing to give it. They see becoming independent of their families as part of their maturation. The Caucasian never does. His strength comes from the lineage, not from his prowess as an individual or his own possessions. This is why the worst punishment he can receive is to be stripped of the family name.

In modern times, resettlement, the greater diversity of opportunity, and occupational migration often unite communities consisting of members of two or more extended families. Neighboring settlements have also merged through growth. In these neighboring settlements, as in the traditional extended family, mutual assistance and moral support continue. Woods, pastures, and arable lands are held in common. In Svanetia in the mountains of Georgia, members of the community are obliged to help the poor families and to take care of orphans without respect to lineage. When someone dies, all the members of the community are obliged to be present, bare-headed, at the burial and to take part in the funeral rites.

One of the most important vestiges of the extended communal family is the kinship terminology. One does not speak of a "relative"; the generic term does not exist. Instead, there are special terms meaning "those born of the son" and "those born of the daughter," i.e., relatives on the father's or mother's side. A boy calls all males of his family "older brother" or "younger brother" depending on their relative age. He calls his mother's male relatives "uncles." In Abkhasia, a woman's children are considered nieces and nephews of not only her own lineage, but also of the entire village from which she came. Age gradations are highly emphasized in Caucasian languages; there are special terms used for addressing women of one's mother's age, men of one's father's age, men of the age of one's older brother, and so forth.

There are many terms for the old extended family commune: "the family with many children," "those living together in one house," "brothers living together," "those who live by one fireplace," and "those who eat out of one pot" are examples. These terms underline family unity. The use of the word "our" also reflects this unity. Thus, "our daughter" may mean a daughter of our lineage. One's sister is the daughter of "our father."

In both the individual family and the family commune, the oldest male possessed the most rights and was the head of the family. His priority and the other age-determined norms for familial interrelationships resulted from the difficulties involved in several generations' living together.

In governing the family, age had great significance—but age would be ignored if the head of the family was unworthy of respect or if he neglected the custom of consulting the other adult members of the family. The fact that he might be removed as the head of the family discouraged his being an autocratic or whimsical despot.

The head of the family still has great influence on all its members, but there are certain changes. He still regulates the family budget, but he can no longer be a dictator. His importance is no longer based on his ownership of the family goods, but on his moral authority and the respect he receives from the rest of the family. It often happens that the head of the family is not the oldest man, but the one who, in the judgment of the family, is best for the position. A colleague told me that in Karabach, Azerbaijan, she found sons heading 6 per cent of the families. In the past, this occurred only when the father was very ill or ancient.

In the past, the whole family was economically dependent on the father, who legally owned everything. Now all the adults, including the women, earn wages. Dependence is therefore moral, ethical, and traditional. In the past, the young bride in her husband's home owned only the dowry she had brought with her. Women's position did not really begin to change until World War II, when women started to do men's work and to earn their own wages.

At the present time the general trend is for the family to break up along generational lines, with sons and their wives establishing separate households after one or more children are born to them. On one Armenian collective farm the young couples were given land for a house on the outskirts of the village. After a while, a street grew up in this region, consisting of some forty households of young people. The villagers called this block "the street without mothers-in-law" since the mother-in-law had previously been an indispensible part of every extended family. Later, however, one elderly woman dubbed it "the street without housekeepers." Since very often both husband and wife work in the fields of the collective at the present time, a mother-in-law would be a welcome and needed addition to the household.

FAMILY COMMITMENT

Despite the break-up of the extended family over the past fifty years, boundless commitment and mutual aid are still characteristic of the Caucasian family. The individual still measures his worth in terms of his ties to each and every one of the members of his family lineage. The more ties he has with different people, the more important he is in his own eyes and in the esteem of others. This is an important point in understanding the respect which the long-living enjoy as heads of large families and of community councils. Each Caucasian may have several hundred persons who are deeply concerned about him and who take responsibility for him. Personal friendships, of course, do develop between relatives, but the basic feeling of security and stability in life comes from this deeply ingrained sense of obligation for each other. As the Abkhasians say, "He who has no relatives will embrace a fence post."

Once, while lecturing in Sukhumi, I asked a student how many relatives she had. "Grandfather says about 500," she replied. A male student then said that his family was not quite so large, consisting of about 300 members. When I told them that I had only a handful of relatives by comparison, they all felt very sorry for me and asked whether I would consider being adopted into some larger family. In the past, families which had lost many male members in wars or epidemics considered themselves weak and vulnerable. Not infrequently they would ask to be adopted by a stronger family.

Americans and Caucasians mean different things by the term "immediate family." We mean only spouses, children, siblings, parents, and sometimes grandparents. When invited to a feast given in honor of an Abkhasian friend of mine who had just graduated from the university, I asked who would be present and was told "the immediate family." When I arrived, there were at least a hundred people in the tiny house. Since it was February and the feast could not be held outdoors, the remainder of the "immediate family" could not be invited.

Everything the extended family owned—arable land, pastures, cattle, and houses—was considered common property. Because of collective ownership, the family was held legally responsible for the actions of each of its members and each individual was held responsible for the actions of his family. When a law was broken, the accused individual had to appear before the village council, accompanied by relatives who could swear to his innocence. If a man was exiled from his village, a few of his closest relatives had to leave with him. This total mutual responsibility naturally required strict control of individual behavior by the family. Anyone guilty of any infraction of the law was punished first by his own family. The head of the family could even order physical punishment if the guilty member was adolescent.

There were precise rules for vindicating oneself before the village council. The number of family witnesses required to testify was in direct proportion to the severity of the crime. For instance, if a man was accused of stealing a stallion, twelve family members were required to swear to his innocence; stealing a mare, required only nine. For a bull, cow, or donkey, six witnesses were needed, and for a lowly goat, only two. In trials for assault, rape, or murder, as many as forty family witnesses might be necessary. If a woman was accused of a crime, her natal family would come forth as witnesses in her behalf. In most areas, women were not permitted to be witnesses. Where they were permitted, two women had to take the place of one man. Collective family responsibility is a concept not even recognized in the laws of the West, except in the case of minors, and even then in a most limited way.

The involvement of the extended family with each of its members made it extremely important to have as many relatives as possible. How can one be alienated in a society where everybody assumes responsibility for everyone else, and where good will and allegiance are infinitely more important than possessions?

Throughout the Caucasus, I was constantly struck by the lack of interest in acquiring possessions. Products and "things" are valued only insofar as they are functional or may promote the comfort of guests. A man may be proud of a good horse or a finely wrought weapon, and a woman may possess some traditional ornaments, but personal possessions are minimal. Most houses are sparsely furnished with little more than simple, long dining tables and chairs for guests. An affluent family might have a sofa or wardrobe but most homes are furnished expressly to accommodate as many guests as possible and the furnishings are clearly aimed at the comfort of guests and ease of entertainment. The most luxurious pieces I saw were in the separate guest houses and not in the family houses.

At a wedding I attended, I was astonished at the great mountain of pillows, blankets, and linen that the bride received as gifts. When I asked how she could use such an enormous quantity of bedding, I was told that of course it was not meant for her personal use, but for the many guests she would naturally expect to receive in her house.

People are wealth in the Caucasus, valued over everything else. One's "wealth" is counted by the number of human relationships one can establish and maintain. One's "success" is measured by the size and strength of the network of loyal and devoted human beings in one's home, extended family, and community.

It is my feeling that the transition to modern collectivization was relatively easy because of the extended family and its innate communal structure. In the memory of most Caucasians is the old extended-family life. For many, collectivization merely reinforced the traditional communal ways.

In small families, which often included only two adult workers, each person had significantly greater responsibilities. The woman was more often called upon to take part in agricultural work, mainly sowing and harvesting. Contradictions about the degree of participation of women in labor can usually be explained by the differences in family form and in the traditionally prescribed divisions of labor.

But no matter what the form of the family, the ubiquitous patriarchal order demanded the subordination of women to men, children to parents, and younger to older.

The head of the family acted as foreman in the family's work. Decisions were made at a family council where women often participated. The power of the father or of the eldest man became more absolute toward the end of the nineteenth century and the beginning of the twentieth. Before that time, in the highly democratic structure of the family and community, he could be removed or replaced in the event of his senility or other incompetence. The loss of this democratic prerogative in most communities probably reflects an attempt to preserve family unity against the effects of industrialization by concentrating more autocratic power in the hands of the "leader."

At the end of the nineteenth century and the beginning of the twentieth, the elder more and more frequently handled family property without anyone else's control, leasing land and selling cattle without consulting the family. Individual members of the family owned only their personal belongings, primarily clothing and, for women, the dowry. All that was acquired by the labor of family members, including the earnings of adult sons, belonged to the head of the family. The departure of married sons depended entirely on his will; a son who left without permission received nothing. A divorced or widowed daughter-in-law, no matter how long she had worked in the family, received nothing except her dowry and part of the bride price. If the division of property took place while the head of the family was still alive, he received a larger portion than did his sons.

Inheritance was regulated by the *shariat,* the Islamic law, and by the *adats,* the traditional law. The *adats* commonly took precedence even among such devout Moslems as the Chechens. Under the *shariat,* one eighth of the property went to the widow; the remainder went to the sons and daughters, but the sons received twice as much as the daughters. In childless families, the wives received a fourth; the remaining three fourths went to the nearest male relatives of the deceased. Under the *adats,* only sons could inherit, one of whom took under his supervision his mother, sisters, and brothers. In the absence of adult sons, a close male relative would take on these responsibilities. This pattern of guardianship was insured by the village council.

Certain groups had *adats* which allowed women to inherit small properties —for example, the Ingush *adats* allowed a single cow. However, the woman did not have the right to dispose of such property independently. Neither the *shariat* nor the *adats* recognized her ability to function and make decisions independently. She was wholly dependent on men—father, brother, or husband. Only at the end of the nineteenth and beginning of the twentieth century, under the influence of Russian law, were there incidents challenging the old feudal patriarchal order. The Yekaterinodarsk People's Court in the mountain region of Daghestan, for example, granted the requests of several women for the fair division of property after the death of their fathers or husbands, giving them custody of their own children.

The head of the family still commands great respect from the other members. Even adult sons try to accommodate themselves to his desires and conduct themselves with great deference in his presence. They do not argue with him nor speak without first being spoken to. They do not sit without permission, smoke, or dress casually in his presence. Younger brothers are obliged to show similar deference to older brothers. One Abkhasian man told me that he never allowed himself even to loosen the collar of his shirt in the presence of his father or older brother. When I asked a Chechen friend why there was such formality between brothers, he replied that this was "cultured" behavior. The Soviets, of course, have put great emphasis on the development of "culture," i.e., socialist values, education, and so forth. It is interesting that my Chechen friend used the same term for the structured decorum of the Caucasus.

A sister shows deference to her brothers, a younger sister-in-law to an elder. My friend Mira, a Georgian ethnographer married to an Abkhasian man, told me that she was once good-naturedly pulled back by her elder sister-in-law when she started to go through a door first. "People will think you have no manners," said her sister-in-law.

In the Caucasus, respect goes hand-in-hand with responsibility. In an extended family, the eldest brother enjoyed a special respect since he was the right-hand man of the head of the family and his most likely successor.

Women, who are excluded from participating in blood feuds and from managing the economy or paying debts, are accorded less respect than are those who take these responsibilities. Responsibility and gift-giving operate inversely, with those younger or of lesser rank receiving gifts from their elders or superiors.

Age deference controlled the order in which sons and daughters were permitted to marry. A younger brother was forbidden to marry earlier than his elder; a younger sister could be married only after her older sister.

Personal relations within the family were controlled by the patriarchal traditions. All members of the family showed absolute allegiance to the head. "The husband," declares the Ossetian *adats,* "is the master and judge of his wife. . . . The husband has the right to punish his wife for disobedience. . . ." The Ingush *adats* demanded that "the wife must not try to teach the husband anything, but must listen to him." Among all Caucasians, the wife must try to please her husband and to show him various signs of respect, such as serving him at meals, taking off his shoes, and washing his feet. The power of the husband over his wife was reinforced by the virtually unilateral right of divorce since the *adats* of most peoples allowed divorce only with the consent of the husband. The *shariat* allowed a husband to expel his wife from the house without explanation, and limited the initiative of a wife to certain defined situations, such as a husband's excessive cruelty, infidelity, or sexual impotence. A divorce initiated by the wife was considered shameful for her and was a rare occurrence. It was also a terrible insult to the husband.

However, a woman enjoyed considerable authority over her children, in particular over her daughters. Among the Chechens, she even had the final say on a daughter's marriage. If she was the "eldest" of a large family, she also had authority over her daughters-in-law, who must accord her obedience and courtesy. Daughters-in-law were required to perform many tasks for their mother-in-law's personal comfort, including combing her hair, washing her feet, and scratching her back. There is a Caucasian song sung by daughters-in-law: "For my beloved mother-in-law, I will make a pillow of thorns, so that she may sleep to her heart's desire." In anger, a mother-in-law might strike her daughter-in-law even though she would never allow her son to do so.

The eldest woman of the family was the mistress of the household and had control over all of the domestic supplies. Among many peoples (the Adygeis, Karchais, Balkarians and others), she alone had the right to go into the pantry.

AVOIDANCE PATTERNS

Familial avoidance patterns, though now modified, were of major importance in the past. Certain members of the family could not be seen together or communicate at all. There are many possible reasons for the development of avoidance patterns. Whatever their origin, they clearly minimized conflict and prevented anger and jealousy between members of a family. The constant interaction of family members required extreme self-control to avoid friction. Singling out one's own child for affection or showing feeling for a husband or wife could easily provoke jealousy in such a communal setting. In the Caucasus, especially among Moslem groups, avoidance was practiced between husband and wife, parents and children, a wife and the relatives of her husband, and a husband and the relatives of his wife.

Married couples were denied the possibility of being alone together in the same room during the daytime, conversing, or eating together, especially when they were still young. They were not to be seen together by older relatives or in public. It was considered reprehensible for a spouse, especially a husband, to display concern for the mate in the presence of outsiders or even to speak to her or him. Spouses were forbidden to address one another by their first names or by the terms "husband" and "wife." Instead, they were to use special third-person terms. It was particularly important not to violate these avoidance patterns in the presence of elderly relatives. To this day, Caucasians consider the public demonstration of emotion to be shameful and indecent. At gatherings, it was often difficult for me to identify couples. Only when I asked would I be told, with some reluctance, who was married to whom.

Avoidance patterns persisted until the time of the Soviets and, to some extent, are still practiced today out of respect for tradition. When I asked a couple to sit next to each other for a photograph, the wife hesitated in embarrassment until her husband indicated his reluctant agreement. "This is against our custom, but if you want to take a picture. . . ." He motioned to her to sit down and I took the picture. On another occasion, I had no difficulty photographing an old couple of 102 sitting next to each other. I learned later that they were not husband and wife, but milk brother and sister, a term meaning that they had been raised by the same wet nurse.

It was always difficult to learn who was related to a whom and to what degree, unless I asked directly. Usually the answer came from friends of mine who knew the family, because a man would always be reluctant to introduce his wife as such and would refer to her as the mother of so-and-so.

Avoidance patterns between parents and children were more rigid for the father than for the mother, especially in the individual family, since the necessity of taking care of young children precluded strict avoidance. In extended families, a mother would initially avoid caring for her own child, leaving this to the other women. Fathers were expected never to pick up or play with their children, any display of paternal feelings being considered indecent. Avoidance decreased somewhat as the child matured, but parent-child relations were always reserved.

The avoidance strictures between parents and their children used to be much more extreme. A father could not call his child by name, speak of it as a boy or girl, or come to the child's assistance even if it were in grave danger. The ethnographer M. Alibokov gave a chilling illustration: At a home Alibokov was visiting, a father went into the stable and found that his little son had been gored by a bull and was still impaled on the bull's horns. He returned to the house and announced, "There, in the stable, a child is crying."

Avoidance between a wife and her husband's relatives mainly involved his older relatives. Some groups forbade her being seen by her father-in-law. In other groups, she was simply forbidden to converse with or look directly at the faces of older in-laws. This avoidance could be relaxed with time, always at the initiative of the older relatives. Among some peoples, a ceremony of acquaintance would end the avoidance between the young bride and the parents of her husband. Among others, the birth of the first child marked the end of avoidance. In Abkhasia, a feast is held where the father-in-law, in the presence of witnesses, offers presents to his son's bride and asks her to speak to him. A story is told in Abkhasia, and in other areas with minor variations, of a man who has given such a feast, but, finding that his daughter-in-law is unbearably talkative, he gives another feast, with many more presents, to persuade her to resume her silence.

The avoidance between a husband and the older members of his wife's family varied in strictness from group to group. The most extreme patterns were to be found among the Cherkessians, the group which also had the most elaborate class system.

According to the old tradition of the Ossetians, the young bride could talk only with the younger people among the family and neighbors and then in a hushed voice. She could not talk at all with the older people or relatives of her husband. She would not even show them her face. For instance, in 1939 in an Ossetian village, Verkhni Ruk, a funeral was held for an old woman. Her older brother-in-law said that for forty years she lived in his family, hard-working, respected by all. "And during all that forty years of her life in our house I see her face for the first time today, but I have never heard her voice because she fulfilled our established tradition."

An Ossetian woman was not allowed to show her face even when she ate. She had to eat after everyone else and rather hurriedly with covered face. With one hand she would lift her veil and with the other she would feed herself. Ossetians were influenced by north Caucasian customs, and the freedom of women found among the Georgians, for instance, was not practiced. In Georgia, both husband and wife were present at the wedding. But among the Ossetians the husband's family changed the daughter-in-law's name when she came to their house or they simply called her daughter-in-law.

Avoidance does not mean that all public demonstrations of all emotion are considered shameful. At a funeral, for example, I saw members of the extended family of the deceased wailing loudly, crying, and scratching at their faces, while his widow sat composed and dry-eyed. Display of feeling is forbidden only to those directly affected by the avoidance patterns. Others are permitted to show affection and concern for one another freely.

Whatever their original justification, however, the avoidance patterns were a heavy burden for women, who were required for long periods of time—sometimes a whole lifetime—to observe these oppressive customs.

A Russian colleague of mine has evidence that avoidance patterns are practiced mostly by women who were married before the Revolution. However, she said, one still finds avoidance here and there "out of respect." For example, Sos, a villager born in 1908, said that his wife, after their marriage in 1928, did not speak to his older brother for twenty years. But his daughter-in-law, who is a university graduate, freely speaks with him and his wife. Today, husbands and wives speak to each other in the presence of others and call one another by their first names, although they still avoid saying "my husband" or "my wife." In Karabach, the wife customarily speaks of her husband as "the man" while the husband refers to his wife as "the daughter of so-and-so." A man born in 1888 told my colleague that he was a member of a lineage which lived in more than one house. He said that when a young husband and wife were left alone with their children in one of the houses, the old people in the next house were terribly contemptuous of such behavior. A woman born in 1904 said that she could not touch her children affectionately in the presence of others and, in fact, could not acknowledge that they were hers.

The persistence of avoidance patterns, many of which are troublesome and not in keeping with contemporary life, apparently serves some important function. It seems to me that avoidance is dictated by the desire not to express preferences for one member of the family over another. It has the effect of reducing sibling rivalry and other competition. Since family membership, not personal attachments, binds one member to another, it is desirable to avoid stressing personal possessiveness. This same idea is stressed linguistically by the survival of archaic forms emphasizing lineage membership and the unity of "our lineage." Avoidance patterns also minimize family disagreements. Resentment, jealousy, and the conflicts which arise naturally from the friction of daily contact are circumvented by simply being ignored. Since avoidance is an institution in both Moslem and Christian areas, it seems clear that it is a pre-Christian, pre-Moslem development.

POSITION OF WOMEN

Since ancient times, the patriarchal principle has dominated life in the Caucasus. Occasional special rights accorded to the mother or mother's brother gave rise to the supposition among Soviet ethnographers that the Caucasians had a stage of matriarchy during their early history, but there are very few shreds of evidence to support this theory. When Islam was introduced, the patriarchal, patrilineal, and patrilocal norms were reinforced by the religious dogma which, in addition to Islamic rules, also enforced some of the local customs, lending them legitimacy. The result was the greatly diminished position of women in the Moslem areas of Daghestan, Azerbaijan, Georgia, and Armenia. In the Christian areas, women were comparatively freer but were still subject to grave limitations.

Islam came to the Caucasus in the seventh and eighth centuries, when Daghestan was conquered by the Arabs. While Moslem doctrine became firmly established in Azerbaijan and Daghestan, it was to some extent modified by pre-Islamic tradition. The amalgamation of the cultures has produced a curious double image of the woman as almost totally subordinate and powerless, and at the same time, strong, courageous and even warlike. Women were to be submissive, their faces covered, their voices not heard, in the Moslem tradition, and yet they were taught to ride horseback, manufacture and use weapons, hunt, and fight the enemy. In the fourteenth-century epic, *Partu Patime,* Tamerlane, the "storm of the universe," who had never suffered a single defeat in his years as a warrior, addresses the heroine of the epic, a simple Lak girl: "The universe has heard my war cry. I have captured kings, won over countries, but I see now for the first time a division in front of me, following a girl-warrior into battle."

We can only speculate on the pre-Islamic roots of this paradox by referring to the numerous myths of the region which celebrate the legendary Amazons. The image of the fighting woman is very old. It is interesting to note the coincidence of these myths in both the Caucasus and Greece.

According to Greek myths and some ancient historians, the Amazon society arose on the shores of the Black Sea and its history is entwined with that of the Scythians. In the fourth volume of his *History,* Herodotus tells of the Greek victory over the Amazons at the River Thermaton in Asia Minor. The Amazons were taken aboard three ships as prisoners of war and sailed back to the Caucasus. During the journey on the open sea, the Amazons, characteristically, killed all the Greek men and, because they did not know the art of navigation, were driven by the wind to Scythia. There they came ashore, captured a herd of horses, and began to plunder the land of the Scythians. The Scythians did not know the invaders or their language, and it was only after they had killed some in battle that they discovered they were warring with women. The Scythians met and decided that rather than kill any more Amazons, they would send their young men to try to woo them. The men pitched their tents in the neighborhood of the Amazons and the two camps soon merged and lived together in harmony. When the Scythians proposed that the women come to live in their society, the Amazons refused, saying they could not get along with Scythian women. If the Scythians wanted them for wives, they must leave their homes and go with the Amazon women. The young Scythians did just that and settled with the Amazons in the vicinity of the Meotian lake. The union of Scythians and Amazons is thought to have created the nation of Savromat. The Savromats and Scythians are the ancestors of present-day Ossetians and other northern Caucasian peoples. The Savromats, Herodotus wrote, continued their distinctive style of life to the time of his *History:* men and women together riding horseback to the hunt or to war and dressing alike. In 66 B.C., Romans under the leadership of Pompey fought a battle with the Georgians on the banks of the River Kura. Georgian women took part in this battle and many were wounded and taken prisoner by the Romans, who were astonished at the great bravery of the native women.

A seventeenth-century Italian missionary, Lamberti, wrote of the women of Georgia and other tribes who took part in war. The Savromat women's participation in war is evidenced in burial mounds dating from the second and third centuries B.C. Archaeological excavations find women buried with war weapons.

Hippocrates (470–376 B.C.) commented that the Savromat women's right breasts were cut off or cauterized, so that all their physical strength would go into the right shoulder and arm. In some other accounts, this enabled them to use the bow more freely. Caucasians think that the custom is related to wearing corsets which bind the breasts. The Caucasian preference for small breasts may have its echo in the Amazon legends.

In the heroic folklore of the Caucasian tribes, there are many tales of brave women. In one of the Nart legends, the chief of a village called on the men from two other villages to aid him in fighting. One village responded but the other did not. The chief ordered that the men of the uncooperative village be put to death. While the women were mourning their dead, one young woman called upon the others to cease mourning and avenge the deaths of their men. For some time they trained in the use of weapons until they were able to fight the other village, defeat it and behead the chief who had ordered the executions.

A Frenchman, Obri de la Mottre (1674–1743), visited the Chercassians in 1712 and observed that the women rode horseback as well as the men and were skilled at hunting with bow and arrow. He suggested that this tradition might be evidence of the historical location of the Amazons in the region, a suggestion much disputed by historians.

Whatever the relation of the Amazon myths to Caucasian life or history, they are worthy of mention because of the tradition which persists in today's Caucasian women and which manifests itself in real ways. One sees, on the one hand, their extreme modesty and retiring manners and on the other hand, their great inner and physical strength. During World War II, although the women were greatly limited in their rights and privileges, especially in Moslem areas, they acted with great strength and independence, taking over all the work that had been done by the men who were fighting on the front, and, later, actually fighting the enemy alongside the men.

After more than fifty years of Soviet law and influence, the legal rights of women in the Caucasus have changed dramatically. Officially, they have complete equality with men. In the cities they are highly visible in academies, libraries, research institutes, and so on. There are many women in the professions, especially medicine. Attitudes, however, are changing much more slowly than the letter of the law would indicate.

Women's transition from the traditional patriarchy to modern Soviet society differed, of course, from region to region. In the Moslem areas, especially among the more religious Shiite Moslems, the transition was accompanied by fierce struggle. In Azerbaijan and Daghestan, where orthodox Moslem tradition was strongest, it was a traumatic and tragic experience for many women.

I had the opportunity to speak at length with Tagira Aleskerova, an Azerbaijanian woman who is head of the Intourist office in Baku. Tagira, an attractive widow in her fifties, spoke without inhibition about growing up in a traditional Moslem household. She showed no resentment or regret about her past, although she remembered Azerbaijanian women of her childhood who attempted to break with the old patriarchal ways and were harshly persecuted and often killed by their families. Despite Soviet law abolishing the wearing of the veil, any Azerbaijanian woman appearing on the streets without her veil was in grave danger of severe punishment and even death at the hands of her own family.

Even after Soviet reforms, Tagira said, women were extremely limited in their human rights and privileges and were expected to be very submissive and obedient. They were forbidden to see, talk with, or have any relationship with men. Girls were married at a very early age to men whom they had never seen before in their lives. When a family had several daughters, they would show the prettiest one to the mother of the intended groom. When the wedding took place, however, the girl behind the veil could very well turn out to be the ugly duckling of the family.

The oldest brother of the husband had the same patriarchal rights and privileges as his father. Strict obedience to him was expected from all the members of the family. In his presence, the wives of his brothers were not supposed to unveil their faces, just as they were expected to conceal their faces from the father-in-law. When a man died, however, his wife became head of the family. A woman who gave birth only to daughters was considered childless, sufficient reason for her husband to take a second wife. Female servants were very often forced to cohabit with their wealthy employer; the mullah readily sanctioned the relationship by reciting a small prayer. On the other hand, a woman practicing any kind of infidelity or premarital relationship was punished severely and her brother, as Tagira expressed it, was expected to "slaughter the sinner," that is, kill the man responsible.

Tagira's experiences in Azerbaijan were no doubt matched by the women of Daghestan, another orthodox Moslem region. There, for instance, women were forbidden by tradition to possess warm overcoats or any other sort of outdoor clothing. In view of the extreme severity of the winters in this high mountainous region, the law effectively kept women prisoners in their homes.

The Communist Party, eager to enlist women for productive work in the late twenties, undertook to provide them with warm coats. Their slogan was "winter coats for mountain women." Once again, everything was done by the women's families to prevent their receiving these gifts. Opposition to the equality of women was the more painful since it came from their own families.

The experience of Abkhasian, Georgian, Chercassian, and Chechen women in adopting Soviet ways was considerably less traumatic because of the more "liberal" Moslemism practiced in these regions. Women here, for instance, did not have to cover their faces. Their traditionally communal society, in which work was shared by everyone, also contributed to a smoother transition to the Soviet system. But even in these less orthodox areas, many old forms remain intact. At banquets, I was often the only woman seated, except when there was a very old woman in the household, in which case the "privilege" of sitting with the men was extended to her.

One feast in Abkhasia was held to celebrate the graduation of a young village woman from the university. As the first Abkhasian woman linguist graduated from the university, she was allowed to sit with me, (although both of us were first required to bow to the elder), but the other female relatives remained apart. The old women who waited on the men's tables at the feast told me that although they accepted the fact that the young people were gradually changing the old patriarchal way of life and even approved of the changes, they could not bring themselves to violate the old customs.

Likewise, among the intelligentsia in Tbilisi, I found that while superficially the new way of life had been accepted almost completely, often the old customs were the real criteria for making judgments of behavior. There is a time lag between culture change and the integration of this change into ethical and emotional life. The Soviet Marxist explanation of this lag in terms of vestigial or atavistic behavior *(perezhitki, ostatki)* overlooks the fact that often the "vestige" rather than the new idea is normative.

Although the struggle for the equal rights and status of women continues in the Caucasus—as it does, indeed, everywhere—it may be said that the overtly destructive elements of the old laws, such as the wearing of the veil and unquestioned authority of the male, are pretty much gone.

The old traditions seem to coexist peacefully with the new freedoms accorded women by Soviet law. Educated women function without conflict in their professions but in the family or village context, they usually observe the traditional rules of etiquette. The desire not to offend old people by breaking the rules of tradition is common among the young, especially when it comes to important crises in life. The desire to bridge modern life and national tradition seems to be very strong in young women and men who are educated and working away from home. They seem to have little desire to be assimilated, to merge with the majority. On the contrary, by performing certain rites and rituals of their ancestors, they manage to keep their national identity, pay respect to their elders, and yet remain modern people.

THE CAUCASIAN WEDDING

The Caucasian wedding is a most joyous, elaborate affair, a high point of social life to be recounted in stories and anecdotes for many years to come. The wedding always takes place in the groom's home, and always at his family's expense. It involves months of preparation, great expense, and heroic labors on the part of the groom's immediate and extended family, his clan, and his neighbors. To provide barrels full of wine, herds of oxen, sheep, calves, and countless chickens to feed the multitude of guests, all relatives as well as invited guests are expected to contribute. A person who fails to bring some offering is considered lacking in pride or self esteem.

A few years ago I was invited to a wedding in an Abkhasian village of the local schoolteacher and a taxi driver—people of obviously modest means. About 1500 people attended. It was necessary to entertain them in shifts. Men and women sat separately at long, narrow tables placed in the courtyard inside an enormously long tent. In spite of the large number of guests, there was no confusion. The best man registered each gift in a book, which the couple is expected to keep for the rest of their lives. Generosity is rated very highly among Caucasians, and a wedding is a time when generosity is most needed.

The bride must not show herself to outsiders before the wedding. An intermediate stage used to provide for the bride's transition from leaving her own family and entering her husband's family. It is considered improper for a bride to come to her marriage bed directly from her family home. Therefore, the bride is brought to her husband's relatives' home as a temporary stopover.

The bride's family provides her with household necessities and gifts for the groom's female relatives, which she distributes promptly upon her arrival. Before the wedding the groom's family is supposed to contribute what was previously known as a bride price, and which nowadays goes under the name of gifts.

Among many traditional Caucasians, the bride's parents and family remain in their home. They do not see their daughter until months after the wedding, when she is well established in her new home.

The wedding celebration goes on for days, everything done with proper consideration for ritual and etiquette. Numerous elected marshals look after the order and make sure that everything runs smoothly.

The real hosts of the wedding are not the groom's parents but the elected *tamadas,* the masters of ceremonies, who keep the flow of oratory running during the feast. A *tamada* must possess the native gift for eloquence and a good memory. He is the key performer at the wedding.

The toast is a traditional oral narrative praising virtues, real or imaginary, of each participant, and it is usually very long. Caucasians like flowery, ornate comparisions in their speeches. With great flourish and eloquence each speaker in turn must express how honored he feels to be called upon to make a toast.

The following is an Armenian wedding toast:

All of us are gathered here on the happy occasion of this wedding—our relations, our neighbors, and our welcome visitors from near and far. This is a great and joyous day. It brings to my mind an ancient and legendary toast which I heard from my great-grandmother, who lived to be one hundred and fifteen. There once was a beautiful apple, not the apple that brought about the downfall of man, but a good apple. God cut it in two, and one half was sent wandering to the right side of the world. The other half was sent to wander on the left side of the world. Both parts of the apple looked upon the people of the earth—on births and deaths, on love and hate, on happiness and tribulation, on success and failure, on all that human life entails. Having seen those human experiences, the two halves turned towards the center of the world, each searching for the other half. When they finally discovered each other, they moved closer and closer, until they joined and became one. So it is with the couple whose union we are celebrating today. They are like the halves of the apple, which searched for one another and at last became one.

Let us drink to their happiness and full life.

THE WEDDING OF MY FRIEND GACAN FROM THE VILLAGE OF KHAIKHI

Gacan is from the Lak village of Khaikhi high in the mountains of Daghestan. Khaikhi has 120 households or, as the natives call them, "chimney smokes." Gacan is a very handsome man of about thirty-two, slim and dark-haired, with a high-school education and agricultural training. Although he is the head of a village collective and has traveled extensively, he says he has never seen anything as entertaining and beautiful as a Lak wedding. He considers his own wedding the most glorious event in his life.

A Lak wedding includes the entire village, regardless of the financial standing of the family. Nobody is invited to the wedding because it is assumed that the whole village will come. Everyone in the village, especially relatives and friends, contributes food and money. The feast, which goes on for three days, requires a lot of food. The male friends of the groom go from home to home collecting chickens. Women bring prepared food in large wooden containers. The mother and relatives of the bride prepare halvah.

During the first day, the entertainment takes place in two homes, the bride's and the groom's. The matchmakers serve the breakfast. The groom sends his representatives to the bride's house to choose the delegation which will bring her to him. The emissaries he sends are served food by the women of the bride's house. After fortifying themselves with fine food and drink, they work out the route of the wedding procession in detail. That evening, accompanied by torchlight and music, the veiled bride is led to the groom's house. The pride of each village demands that it not part lightly with its brides. The young people of the bride's village "cut the road" to delay her departure. That is, they arrange games on what is really a narrow path to create obstacles. The old people go through the motions of reasoning with the young people not to be overzealous but to permit the procession to continue. The trip which ordinarily takes about fifteen minutes is stretched out to four or five hours.

The procession arrives at last at the groom's house and the wedding feast begins. Although the affair appears to be spontaneous, it is really very carefully planned. The place of honor is given to the old people and dinner is sent to the homes of those who could not attend. The old people sit at a separate table and select their own *tamada* (the host of the table). The role of the "whitebeards" at the wedding is to grace the event since they are the most respected in the community. They also mediate disputes and give advice whenever asked. It is beneath their dignity to give advice without being asked. While it is the prerogative of young people on specified occasions to be exuberant, the old must act with moderation after careful thought, and they are able to keep the young people in check. As at all Caucasian banquets, the head *tamada,* chosen by the whole village, selects the best dishes and sends them to the table of the elders who are usually eighty or older.

The head *tamada* selects functionaries whose duty it is to keep things in order and running smoothly. He also selects someone who knows folk medicine to be the doctor of the wedding and to administer first aid if it is needed.

When a man brings a gift—a live sheep or goat—he puts it on his shoulders and dances before the guests. Each woman brings a gift on a platter which she carries on her head as she dances in front of all the guests. The man chosen to be in charge of the gifts loudly announces the name of the husband or brother of the woman who brings the gift. She cannot give in her own name.

The women sit apart from the men. The main functions of the wedding are carried out by the men. After the dinner at the groom's home, the guests go to the spring to drink water, dance, talk, and sing until it is time to go to the *shurna.*

The *shurna* is a reception given by the parents of the bride. The traditional dish is a mutton bouillon mixed with pickle sauce. This is considered a good dish for sobering up after drinking, but more drinks are served at the *shurna.*

After this, the bride and groom are left in the house of the groom and the marriage is consummated. In the past, it was a point of honor for the bride to put as many obstacles as possible in the way of her new husband. She would actually fight him very hard. When she was overpowered, the husband untied the knots she had tied in her clothing. Exercising his patience was considered a great value. Thus she demonstrated her modesty and the importance of her virginity and he manifested his masculinity by his restraint and patience.

The matchmaker takes up his position at the door of the bridal chamber to guard the couple's privacy. When the marriage is consummated, the groom knocks on the door, and the matchmaker announces the happy news to the guests who respond with joyful shouts, laughter, music, dancing, and gun shots.

If the bride is discovered not to be a virgin, the husband may throw her out of the window. When I expressed surprise and horror, Gacan said that she was never thrown from higher than the ground floor. Shame, not physical pain, is the worst damage inflicted. But of course, said Gacan with a gleam in his eye, that did not happen to his bride.

On the third day, guests who have come from neighboring villages are fed and given gifts of halvah, meat, bread, and fruit. And so the wedding ends.

The Laks are Moslems of the Sunni order and in the past a mullah was invited to perform the marriage ceremony. Every village had a mosque and a mullah. No mosques remain; either they have been razed or are used as movie theaters. Now the marriage is registered in the village soviet. But the old customs have not been forgotten; they have simply become traditions, as happens in a great many other places in the Soviet Union.

As I listened to Gacan telling me the story of his wedding with pride and affection, so careful not to skip a single step in the sequence, I wondered what exactly it was that made Gacan so devoted to his traditions. Gacan is a Communist, well aware of progress in a Marxist sense, yet so unashamedly devoted to the survival of the old order.

It occured to me that it might be the smallness of the Lak group; they number only 70,000. Constant migration out of the area has reduced their number greatly. They are skilled laborers, jewelers, coppersmiths, tradesmen, masons, pastry cooks, cobblers, and acrobats. They may feel that in order not to be smothered by larger neighboring tribes they must observe their customs and speak their native language. Perhaps in the past they were a larger and more important group. Arabic sources of the ninth and tenth centuries mention them as native to the area. Now the Lak language has five dialects, used in speaking and writing. Writing started to flourish only after the Revolution when an alphabet was devised for them. Before that a little was written in Arabic script.

A friend of mine told me about a Nogai wedding she attended in a village in the northern Caucasus. The couple had been married for some months already. The wife was Russian and her husband was a university-educated Nogaj. They lived in the city, but had returned to the village for a traditional wedding. The bride, being unfamiliar with the customs, did not strictly abide by them. Instead of standing silent and veiled in a corner while the festivities proceeded, she became nervous and seized her husband's arm and would not let him go during the whole evening. The husband, seeing his bride pale and shaken, kissed her reassuringly a few times and spoke endearing words to her. All this his mother surveyed with horror and indignation. As she recounted the bizarre carryings-on of her son and his wife, each item was followed by "and I was so insulted." The breaking of the tradition was viewed by the mother as a deep personal insult. The behavior was not viewed as a breach of religious taboos and therefore no sacred sanction was involved. It was a breach of custom and therefore insulting to older people. This society was held together by customs, not religion.

THE RELATIONSHIP BETWEEN GENERATIONS

It was a warm spring day when we visited the small Georgian village of Ananuri, where I was to search out and interview some longevous people. The head of the Gerontological Institute in Tbilisi had given me a list of elderly people living in the village. As we approached our destination, I went over the names and ages of the people I was to meet. Since it was almost noon and we had left Tbilisi by car at six o'clock in the morning, I wondered aloud whether there would be an inn or some collective farm cafeteria where we could have something to eat. My companion, a fifty-year-old retired medical doctor, and the driver, a young man, were both Georgians. They smiled reassuringly at me and said, "No need to look for restaurants—we'll be fed in every home we enter. You'll see. No Georgian family would let a guest go without offering food and drink." Indeed before the day was over we had been wined and dined in quite a few homes in the village.

My list of longevous people was about three years old. Four of the people on the list had passed away, while five had reached the one-hundred-year mark. It turned out that there were even more longevous people in the village than the list had indicated.

It was Sunday, and many people were out walking. Since more complete information can be obtained when the whole family is together, we had chosen Sunday for our interviews.

We stopped in front of a house and the driver told me that he personally knew the woman sitting on the ground to be 104 years old. She appeared to be sitting directly on the ground, though on closer examination a rug was visible. She was not on my list but nevertheless I decided to interview her. As we climbed out of the car, she quickly glanced up at us and went back to her work. She was stripping the down from feathers, apparently for use in a quilt. When my driver asked her in Georgian whether she would stop for a moment to talk with us, she replied that she was busy preparing her great-granddaughter's dowry and had no time. The pressing urgency of her work appeared all the more surprising when her great-granddaughter turned up—a little twelve-year-old.

The girl looked at us and then went over and put her arms around her great-grandmother. I asked when she was getting married. She laughed and said, "Of course I'm not getting married right away. I am at school now, but someday I will, and so my great-grandmother is preparing." She seemed to accept the fact that her great-grandmother was anxious and concerned about her dowry and that time played no part in her planning. Her great-grand-mother, likewise, accepted the fact that the girl was still at school and would not be getting married soon. Attitudes that would have seemed mutually contradictory in the West were here accepted without any objections or hostility. In other words, they respected the thoughts and desires of each other and accommodated themselves without causing any friction.

The harmony and rapport between the little girl and her great-grand-mother reflect a continuity of values which transcends time and change. There is no "communications gap," despite the changes brought about by industrialization. In our own society, the very meaning of words changes from one generation to the next, sometimes even sooner. A twelve-year-old and an eighty-year-old must speak to each other across a great chasm of shifting values and meanings and often might well be speaking different languages. No such confusion exists in the stable society we are describing. The belief, so widespread in our modern world, that all things new are good, and all things old are valueless, has not even begun to make inroads there. The little girl and her great-grandmother speak the same language because they share the same values. The harmony and lack of tension between genera-tions may be due in part to the fact that parents do not try to live through their children. They do not, for instance, press them to accomplish things that they might like to do themselves but cannot. Contentment is, in any case, more highly valued than success.

The 104-year-old woman claimed that she was sitting on a rug on the ground because it was easier to work that way. I was none too warm in my winter coat, and I asked her whether she would not catch cold. She laughed and said in Georgian, "What funny ideas you have! I never catch cold, and besides, why should one catch cold sitting in the sun?" I took a few snapshots of her, but when I begged her to raise her head so that her face could be seen, she replied that she had no time, and besides, what's so important about taking a photograph? Anyway, there would be plenty of time for me to look at her, since we were going to be invited to the house of her grandson.

A few minutes later the little girl's father emerged from the house and asked us in. My companion, the driver, and I entered, and in a few minutes the family and a few neighbors had gathered around the table. In all areas of the Caucasus, when a visitor arrives neighbors immediately come to in-quire whether they can provide food or help with the work. I therefore found it difficult to distinguish between neighbors and members of the family.

The neighbors were eager to answer questions, especially the elderly people who remembered things that were unfamiliar to the young. I was curious how much and what kind of work the old woman did, as she seemed to be the oldest member of the household. I was told that she sewed beautifully and also knitted sweaters. In fact, the girl was wearing a lovely sweater that her great-grandmother had made for her. I asked whether the old woman needed glasses to sew. The answer was that she neither needs nor has them. She also does some cooking and feels generally responsible for the household, although it is run by the wife of her grandson. She slept, I was told, in the living room, the largest and best ventilated room in the house, in a large comfortable bed. Nobody in the house would think of coming in and disturbing her until she was awake. However, she arose early. I was interested in her working habits and whether she tired after several hours of working. She said there was no reason for her to be tired by work she knows and likes, but she did rest during the day whenever she felt tired. Her day follows a very definite, rhythmic pattern: she rises at the same hour each day, works, rests, and eats at the same times. The chemistry of her body and its biological functioning seem to have adapted to this pattern.

No fuss is made over great age. The old people are always busy. During my wanderings in the Caucasus I never encountered an old woman or an old man sitting idle, although the younger folks seemed better able to enjoy idleness. The members of the family take it for granted that old people want to work. Occasionally, merely as a gesture, they may try to restrain their great-grandparents, but the old people know that they are perfectly capable of assuming various responsibilities in the large household.

CHILDREN

In all Caucasians, the desire for children is great, especially for boys to perpetuate the family line. If a wife is barren or bears only girls she can be divorced. It is not even considered that the man might be the cause. When a divorce does take place, the children usually stay with the father.

Although children are considered a great blessing, bringing happiness to the household, a strict upbringing is the rule. Indeed, a family incurs sharp criticism if it is felt that they give their children too much freedom—an indication that they do not care as much for their children as they should. Obviously, it takes more time and effort to supervise children strictly. Permissiveness is thought to spoil children, make them irresponsible, and retard their growing up.

The family size considered desirable varies according to region. In Azerbaijan, the number of children, as a rule, is very large. In Abkhasia, where people marry much later, the pattern favors small families. The Abkhasians compensate by extending the family to include ritual friends, acquaintances, or neighbors who come into some meaningful contact with them. Hence their family membership is large. For example, the midwife who delivers a child becomes a member of the family when she cuts the umbilical cord. The first time I was to visit Abkhasia, I was asked in Moscow if I had relatives there, because, they said, all Abkhasians were related. Sure enough, during the course of my visit, I received an offer to be "adopted" by an Abkhasian family.

The birth of a child is celebrated by the entire patronymic group, but the relatives on the mother's side also play an important role in the feasting. The number of participants depends on the social status of the family. While most peasants have rather modest feasts, the well-to-do arrange races with prizes in honor of the male child, along with sumptuous meals, dancing, singing, and games. In the northern areas a national drink, *buza,* is prepared from fermented millet. In "the tying of the red cheese" a tall pole is erected with a firm crosspiece from which is suspended an ordinary, round, smoked cheese. Next to it is attached a well-greased leather rope, which the young men of the village try to climb to reach the cheese. Whoever reaches the top first and bites off a piece of cheese receives a special prize.

In some villages it was customary to announce the birth of a boy by flying a red flag on the roof of the house so blessed. Villagers passing by and even strangers would stop at the house to congratulate the happy grandmother and grandfather, but never the parents, who are, according to custom, not allowed to acknowledge parenthood. The celebration is arranged not by the parents, but by the grandparents, or, in their absence, by older aunts and uncles. Through intermediaries, the parents are told of the day of celebration.

Caucasian parents have often been characterized as remote and unaffectionate toward their children. The lack of outward, public manifestations of affection has been taken as coldness. For a father to handle or fondle his own children, or even to call them by name, is considered unmanly. This avoidance pattern, however, applies only to one's own offspring; it is entirely permissible to show affection to the children of friends. Dr. Louis Luzbetak considers these avoidance patterns a reflection of the low status of women in Caucasian society; affection to children is associated with femininity. However, since avoidance patterns bind the women as well as the men, it seems an unlikely explanation. Others explain the avoidance patterns in terms of the group marriage.

It seems likely to me that avoidance is an exercise in the self-restraint necessary in a spartan, military-type society. Caucasian life for countless generations was characterized by constant warring, blood feuds, and inter-group rivalry. The military virtues of bravery, emotional self-restraint, and resourcefulness were highly prized. Since customs often linger long after the conditions which created them have disappeared, especially in integrated, stable societies, the avoidance patterns are still retained.

Prohibitions on the demonstration of affection to one's own children is intended to make them stronger and tougher. Yet the children must be made to know that their parents have their best interests at heart and to realize that is necessary for their parents to uphold the accepted values and codes of behavior.

ATALYK

Atalyk is the Turkish name given an ancient Caucasian child-rearing custom. Small children and infants are sent away from home to be brought up by another family. Although there are many interesting historical and ethnographic speculations about the reasons for this institution, it seems to me very much of a piece with the Caucasian ideal of a spartan upbringing to toughen the child. Rearing a child in a family other than his own effectively eliminates the possibility of parental partiality.

Atalyk persisted well beyond the first quarter of the twentieth century and seemed to fill a number of cultural needs. Many adults in present-day Caucasian society were brought up by foster parents, and I spoke to many who retain deep attachments to their foster-parents and foster-siblings. Because of historical interest and because it was so important in the social and political structure of the Caucasian people, many Russian travelers and ethnographers have described the custom.

Atalyk was practiced by the feudal nobility more than by the lower classes, and even when it had died out elsewhere, it continued for a long time in noble families. It was unthinkable for them to bring up a child in their own home. The custom was to place the children in a home of lower socioeconomic status than that of the noble household, and in another village. The foster-households, in turn, would seek out a family lower than themselves with which to place their own children. The peasants, if they desired to follow *atalyk* custom, could only give children to each other.

Although feudalism was very weak in the Caucasus, the Cherkessians developed a feudal nobility with a strong, clear-cut class system. *Atalyk* was obligatory for them. When a woman of an important family was pregnant, a number of possible *atalyk* families were evaluated and considered. The real mother was allowed to see the baby only once during its childhood, and the father not at all. Since the foster-child and the children in the *atalyk* household would be considered brothers and sisters, *atalyk* established a truly meaningful relationship between the two families which included help and affection on all levels. Sometimes in the course of a blood feud, a baby was stolen by one of the rival families. They reared the child to adulthood and then returned it to its own family, whereupon both families, having a child in common, would have to make peace.

The wife of the *atalyk* family was wet nurse and foster-mother. She cared for the infant for two or three years or until the nursing period was over. Then, if the child was a boy, he would come under the supervision of the foster-father, who would educate him in manners and speech and the skills of hunting and war. Periodically, the foster-parents honored their foster-child with a celebration to which they invited their own entire village, but not that of the real parents. The guests were supposed to bring presents—perhaps a horse or a dagger, if the child was a boy. The parties marked important events, such as the child's first steps and first haircut, and involved the entire village in the upbringing of the child.

During the years the child lived with the *atalyk* family, he played, ate, slept, exercised, and worked with the other children of the family. It often happened that a child was given to a family of another tribe to establish peaceful relations. The child was kept almost as a hostage to insure the peace.

At the age of fourteen or fifteen, the child was considered a man or woman, capable of adult work, and the foster-parents informed the real parents that the child was ready to return. A great feast was organized to welcome him or her home.

More often he felt closer to the *atalyk* family than to his own. When there was an argument between the real and the *atalyk* father, the boy would always take the part of the *atalyk* father, but such a situation was rare since the real father was in a higher position. In the past, if one family was involved in a blood feud, it was absolutely required that the other family also take part.

Remuneration for the years of tutoring and support was never money but something like cattle or a piece of land, depending on the wealth of the parent family. The gifts had to be very substantial. On the other hand, the *atalyk* family was expected to bring gifts and food to help feed the many guests at the celebration of the child's return.

Atalyk served two important purposes besides producing strong, independent individuals: (1) It cut across class lines and established a personality which may be described as the Caucasian personality, and, (2), it established

intertribal familial alliances of great economic, social and political importance. It was another means of extending the family and creating a supportive
structure of human relationships.

Although *atalyk* is no longer practiced, its values and methods of child-
rearing remain essentially intact. Most of the adults and all of the old people
in Caucasian society today were reared in the traditions embodied in the
atalyk and have carried them into the present. Although certain concessions
are made to modern technology in matters of food, clothing, shelter, and
medical care, they are peripheral to the essentially unchanged emphasis on
the priority of human relationships over material concerns. The single factor
which most effectively perpetuates the traditions is the great deference and
respect still accorded to parents and old people by the great majority of the
young. Of course, the presence of many long-lived people reinforces these
attitudes.

For the inculcation of traditional values, certain behavior patterns must,
of course, be established during infancy and childhood. Physical contact
between parents and children is kept to a minimum, in keeping with the
avoidance patterns. Contact between mother and child can take place only
in the parents' bedroom, out of sight of older relatives.

For the first year the infant is strapped into a wooden rocking cradle with
openings at the bottom to allow urine to flow out. Swaddling is tight and
constricting. He is taken out of the cradle no more than three or four times
during the day, but sleeps with his mother at night. Breast-feeding usually
continues for the first year and a half. At six to eight months, he is started
on animal milk and porridge, and at one year he begins to eat the same food
as adults, though breast-feeding may continue in some cases for three or more
years.

Among the Moslems, the final ritual of the early years of a boy's life is
circumcision, when he is about four. Since in many regions circumcision was
not performed by natives but by traveling Daghestanians, the ritual was often
observed somewhat earlier or later, depending on when the visiting specialist
appeared.

Both boys and girls are taught from an early age to respect and show
courtesy to their elders and to master the many and complex rules of Caucasian etiquette. A child becomes responsible for his actions at the age of seven.
Until that time, his parents are held responsible for his behavior.

In most families of the Northern Caucasus, differences in the treatment of
boys and girls begin at six to eight years. Until then, regardless of sex,
children run around and play together, but cannot bathe in the river at the

same time. Little girls begin to be differentiated earlier than boys. They are kept at home more and, as a rule, begin working earlier than boys. Girls as young as six to eight years have to take care of the younger children and serve the older ones. They are taught to clean the house and prepare food. They also learn the many cottage skills.

Children sleep in their parents' rooms until the age of ten or twelve. Then the boys are sent to sleep in the guest room. The girls, if possible, are given separate rooms. At this point, children often receive a new and more complete set of clothes. Girls are no longer allowed to leave the house alone, go out after dark, remain alone, or converse alone with an outside boy.

The education of boys, which until this time has been primarily in the hands of women, is now taken over by the men who begin to include them in their work. Adolescent boys become herdsmen and cattle drivers. They help care for livestock, cut firewood, tie and carry hay, participate in harvests, and learn the trades of men. In keeping with the patriarcho-feudal way of life in the Northern Caucasus, they also learn to ride and use firearms, and are taught to love work and discipline, as well as endurance and bravery. Chechen men, for example, encourage the fights of adolescent boys; the winners are praised and the losers are teased.

Adolescent girls are also taught to ride horseback, but playing musical instruments and dancing are stressed to a greater extent.

At fifteen or sixteen, a youth is already capable of men's work, carries a weapon, participates in horse racing, and is recognized by the traditional law as an adult. A girl is adult at the fourteen or fifteen. She is then eligible for marriage and can perform all of a woman's tasks.

Caucasian parents regard the rearing of children strong in body and spirit as their prime duty. Great importance is given to healthy physical development. The very nature of the environment promotes energetic physical activity. Children often walk several miles to school each day, especially in areas where homesteads are scattered or where there is one school serving several villages. Since most of the settlements in mountain regions are on slopes, there is constant walking up and down steep mountain paths. Men, women, and children do not mind walking long distances to fetch spring water, which is considered especially healthful. Going to the fields of the collective farm, visiting friends, and going to the movies is all done on foot. Horses are still used widely for traveling longer distances, although cars have become more common in recent times.

A generation or two ago in the United States, children thought nothing of walking to school; children in rural areas covered many miles a day. It was an accepted way of life. Today, however, children are driven to and from school by their mothers or a car pool, or else take school buses or public transportation. Self-locomotion is just about obsolete.

Caucasian boys learn horseback riding, stone-throwing, wrestling, running, running on stilts, archery, pole-vaulting across barriers, rock-climbing, skiing, and competitive running and riding games. They develop balance by walking on poles laid across crevices or streams.

Most children's games are collective. Wrestling may be one-to-one, but often a few smaller boys will wrestle with an older one. It is not considered shameful to lose in wrestling.

Although not all Caucasian groups observe elaborate rites of passage into adulthood, almost all test the skills and physical fitness of young boys at puberty. Often a special committee of old people presides over the tests of skill, which everyone must pass in order to be considered an adult. Among the most valued attributes are grace, strength, speed, horsemanship, and the use of weapons. Physical skill is not enough in itself but must be set within the context of gracious human relations; a young man is also judged on his intelligence, quick wit, and knowledge of traditions, courtesy, etiquette, and the rituals of hospitality. In Daghestan, a young horseman must know that when he leaves the home of his host he must walk his horse slowly to the edge of the village before he gallops away in a cloud of dust.

Despite other differences, there seems to be a common agreement among Caucasians on what constitutes "virtue" in men and women. Physically, the ideal Caucasian woman is slim, with small waist, hips, breasts, feet, and hands. Her forehead should be high. Her stature is not so important. Expressive eyes are appreciated since a woman does not speak flirtatiously. She must show modesty and not look directly at a man. The most valued quality is grace. From an early age both boys and girls are taught good coordination so that as adults they move rhythmically, like dancers. Mountain people have a distinct and graceful gait, walking with small, fast steps. Clumsiness is almost worse than stupidity. Cleverness is appreciated but sensitivity to other people is essential. Interacting with so many individuals of different degrees of relationship requires a great deal of tact and feeling.

Although school is now compulsory and girls go to school until the age of seventeen, their status in the family is not changed by education. Their attitude toward parents and siblings still conforms to traditional standards. They are expected to be obedient, respectful, and more industrious than men.

There are basic housekeeping skills without which no girl would be allowed to marry.

She should be able to dance gracefully at weddings and other festivities. Since young Caucasian girls are expected to be shy and modest, dancing is the only means of self-expression.

For men, slenderness and grace are as necessary as for women. Horseback riding, a highly developed art, expresses masculinity. Old men limit their riding to displays of unusual skill—sliding under the horse's belly, for example.

Men select their vocations when they finish school at seventeen.

A man should be courageous, responsible, loyal, and truthful—"a man of his word." Caucasians must not break a promise—even one made for them by their parents. A person disgraces both himself and his family by breaking a promise and often provokes revenge.

"A man who controls his speech owns the village," say the Abkhasians. "Human beings learn to talk in two years, but need sixty years to hold their tongues," say the Daghestinians. Another saying is, "When you told me for the first time, I believed you; when you repeated yourself the second time I was in doubt; but when you repeated yourself the third time I knew you were lying."

Self-discipline and self-control are required of both men and women from a very early age. The structured, predictable behavior and the mechanisms for dealing with disappointment or disaster minimize conflict and stress. When faced with a difficult situation, a Caucasian can generally reconcile himself to it more readily than a Westerner because he can draw upon the many societal structures available to him for a solution, and on his own deeply ingrained self-discipline.

The impersonal code that old and young obey functions effectively in the Caucasus. As the key concepts in upbringing it requires pride and dignity. Eating and speaking, walking and even dying must be done with dignity. Psychological and physiological demands are acknowledged only as they fit into the recognized scheme of custom and behavior.

With all the restraints demanded and practiced in everyday life, some relief is required. There are many socially sanctioned outbursts that provide the people with occasional safety-valves, like horse racing, sports, dancing, and singing.

STRESS AND CHILD-REARING

Caucasian longevity has been attributed to lack of stress. This is naive and simplistic, since no human being can always avoid stress. Stress is built into the physical and spiritual life of all people, the Caucasians no less than others. Indeed, for countless generations Caucasian life was characterized by constant warring, blood feuds, intergroup rivalries, and periodic epidemics, as well as the rigors of their rocky, mountainous environment and a thicket of restrictive rules.

The Caucasians do not avoid stress but deal with it. They have developed many mechanisms—physical, psychological, and symbolic—which enable them to face and resolve situations which create stress. The children, for example, are taught that excuses are not acceptable; they must look for a solution or an option. When something is broken, it must be mended—whether it be a pot or a human relationship. Rather than apologizing for an error or misstep, one corrects it. Petty quarreling and arguments are considered unnecessary irritations and a waste of energy.

Soviet society stresses the prime importance of formal education. The Caucasians acknowledge its importance, but rank it below the military virtues of bravery, emotional self-restraint, and resourcefulness—values developed in the past and still cherished in the present.

When children need help they turn first to their siblings and playmates. In playing, climbing, and riding, they are taught not to be afraid of danger, but rather to be aware of it and to face it when necessary.

Consistency and stoicism from earliest childhood prepare Caucasians to bear the stresses of poverty, warfare, and natural accidents without unnecessary emotional or physical trauma. They can take severe blows without going to pieces, and they have developed a peculiar optimism, in spite of centuries of economic hardship and uncertainty.

One would expect to find a certain degree of fatalism among Moslems, but it is surprisingly absent from Caucasian Moslems. They consider their fate to be primarily self-determined, but at the same time they are able to make peace with the inevitable. They do not passively accept what befalls them, but neither do they struggle uselessly against things which cannot be changed. A certain harmony with nature and the environment is achieved through self-control rather than fatalism.

The stoic upbringing, which starts in infancy, instills respect, obedience, and endurance. Since the home often holds as many as five generations, there is no dearth of examples of correct conduct. The child is immersed in an atmosphere where what is expected is absolutely clear and is reinforced by virtually every member of the community. It is assumed that the child will internalize the same values.

A child is never beaten, scolded, or humiliated in front of others, since he cannot have self-discipline if his spirit is broken. My Chechen friend said that if children were punished physically they would "feel themselves slaves" and lose their pride. Although some groups, such as the Azerbaijanians, physically punish their children in private—but never on the face since it is publicly visible—others, like the Abkhasians, never beat or humiliate their children. Fostering pride is central to the upbringing of children in the Caucasus. Ridicule is not used as a pedagogical tool. Scorn and rejection are reserved to punish failure in family morals, not failure to achieve.

Parental respect for the privacy and physical autonomy of children partially accounts for the lack of resentment between generations. I never heard a parent urge a child to eat or put on more clothing, or question him about his excretory functions.

Little Chechen boys are taught to decline a favorite food, sometimes for an entire week, "for the sake of discipline." To be taught to master his fears, a five-year-old boy may be sent to a cemetery or deserted mill at night and required to bring back proof that he has been there. With age the difficulty of the tasks increase. Children are expected to be contemptuous of fear and pain. The process that begins by seating a three-week-old infant on a saddle leads to such feats as walking on hot coals in adulthood.

To show emotions means to lose self-control. This idea is projected into their folklore. In the Nart epic there are no descriptions of emotional states. Anger, sorrow, and other feelings are shown only through people's actions. For example, in one of the episodes the father discovers that through a fatal mistake he has killed his only son. "The father grabs the iron ceiling beam and bends it upward," says the narrative. "He then flings himself on the iron bed which buckles under him."

In another episode, Sasrykva's mother is annoyed with him. This is how her anger is pictured: "She sat down with force on the iron bench and broke it. With her head she gave a smashing blow to the ceiling beam."

One day the Narts were dividing their war spoils. When they refused to give Sasrykva an equal share, "He struck the ceiling with his head and the roof of the house where the Narts lived came down. With his hand, he hit the wall and the wall crumbled."

Children listen in silence at meetings to learn eloquence, a very important virtue. Oratory is cultivated but not talkativeness, especially in boys. "Teeth were given us to hold back the words on the tip of our tongues," say the Chechens. Once a word is given, however, it must be kept. "A word is like a dagger—it should not be taken out of the scabbard without reason."

Discipline, as conceived by the Caucasians, is obedience not to others but to internalized standards which govern the manifestation of feelings and impulses and the satisfaction of needs. Real manliness is self-control, not the possession of clothing, wealth, or women. Bravery does not mean not knowing fear; it means mastering fear.

An impersonal code reduces intergenerational conflict since authority figures are guardians of the code, not merely willful, whimsical, and arbitrary. The Eskimos consider breaking a tabu a sign of strength, since authority is seen as autocratic and personal. The Caucasians, however, view a breach of cultural norms as weakness, because their code is objective, absolute, and impersonal.

REPRESSION AND SELF-CONTROL

Western psychologists since Freud have generally viewed repression and alienation as ineluctable consequences of modern society. In *Civilization and Its Discontents* Freud sees an inevitable incongruity between human instinctual drives and the bounds imposed by society. The human condition is thus inherently tragic. R.D. Laing also sees a conflict between the social self and the phantasy self which feels the real, antisocial desires. The existentialists also generally subscribe to the idea of the individual's irreducible alienation in modern society.

In traditional, integrated cultures, however, self-control and self-discipline are matters of habit which do not require the suppression of natural drives so much as their modification. There is no contradiction between one's socially modified desires and one's "real" desires.

This view of self-control through habit, prevalent in the highly integrated Caucasian culture, is expressed by Aristotle in his *Nichomachean Ethics:* one behaves morally correctly out of habit; one's character is one's habitual behavior. There is no recourse to the idea of repression, because there is no contradiction between habitual behavior and real motivation.

Sex, for instance, is guiltless and unrepressed. It is neither projected nor sublimated into work, art, or religious-mystical passion. It is not an evil to be driven from one's thoughts, but a pleasure to be regulated for the sake of health, and it improves with age—like a good wine.

It is my feeling that Caucasian longevity is not the result of freedom from stress, but of dealing with individual stress in a societal structure sustained by inner consistent values which create a biological and spiritual rhythm. No energy is lost in attempting to reconcile elements alien to the established patterns of life. In this respect Caucasian society is conflict-free and noncompetitive. Men and women are judged by the quality of their personal relationships. Harmony is valued over wealth, status, or achievement.

BLOOD FEUDS

The ancient Caucasian tradition of the blood feud demonstrates both the solidarity of the family commune and the formal structure of the society, as well as the stress-reducing mechanisms inherent in the structure. Family unity was at the root of the vicious circle of the blood feud. While cases of intrafamilial murder—a man killing his son or brother, for example—were adjudicated by the head of the family, a murder outside the family invariably resulted in a blood feud. Intrafamilial murders, where "the dog devours his own milk" in the words of an Ingush proverb, were, however, very infrequent. In other cultures the vast majority of homicides are intrafamilial, but the Caucasian family is so tightly knit that such crimes are almost unheard of.

If a murderer desired reconciliation with the family of his victim, he could hide near their homestead until the appropriate moment and then run forward and put his mouth to the breast of the "old woman" of the clan, thereby signaling his desire to become a milk relative and to end the hostilities. Then no one would be permitted to touch him, since milk relations were considered stronger even than blood relations. Marriage between the two warring clans could also bring about a truce. Thus, family solidarity both created the problem of the blood feud and provided for its solution.

Among different groups the blood feuds took different forms. Among Chechen and Ingush groups, the relatives of the deceased would form a band and travel "in war" to the home of the murderer. The besieged clan would take refuge in its battle tower. This "war" was often waged only in a formal sense, since the besieged feared to kill another of their foe and aggravate the feud. The death of one of the besieged, on the other hand, might effect some sort of reconciliation. In the nineteenth century, the murderer might buy the right to travel unimpeded on his own farm for a certain ransom, usually paid in bulls. In the Middle Ages, however, the price of blood was blood; the avenging blow would eventually be struck. Sometimes whole families would be captured and sold as slaves and their land and cattle plundered. In areas where large-scale blood feuds were waged, such as Checheno-Ingushetia, the entire life-style was changed by the large war towers built for defense of the clan. Migrations of entire families to escape revenge were also common.

According to common law of the Daghestanians, if a man grew rich and did not want to be responsible for the actions of his relatives, he could give up relationship performing the special ritual of separation with the permission of the council.

Another decree permitted relatives to take their kinsman's life in order to escape responsibility for his criminal actions.

Among other peoples—the Abkhasians and Svans, for example—the blood feud was carried on by individuals, with the closest male relative of the deceased taking responsibility for revenge.

Women, it should be noted, played only passive roles in blood feuds, serving as frequent causes for the violence. As one proverb phrased it, "Blood which flows because of a woman never ceases." The Abkhasian term for blood feud, "the tail of a woman," expresses the same idea.

The blood, in fact, often did continue to flow for generations, although participants in the feuds might not even remember who had committed the original crime. The reason for the mechanical continuation of the blood feuds is to be found, once again, in the Caucasians' rigid concept of honor. Children were brought up with the idea that revenge is the only honorable response to an injury. Although Caucasians generally have a good sense of humor, even a small boy would not tolerate anyone's touching his hat, even in fun. Blood revenge was thus a sacred duty, totally independent of emotion or inclination.

A good illustration of the unemotional attitude toward violent revenge is a story told to me by an ethnographer at the Academy of Sciences in Moscow. A Svan man had committed a murder for which he had been sentenced to eight years in prison. When the ethnographer asked the villagers about the man's character, they could not praise him highly enough; he was considered a fine worker and brave fighter. But when they were asked how they would relate to the man after his return, they replied, quite matter-of-factly, "We will kill him." His death was regarded as a mechanical necessity in spite of his admitted virtues.

The mechanical nature of the blood feud can be seen in another story about the Svans—a laconic, isolated, and highly parochial people of the mountains of Georgia—which was told to me by a Georgian anthropologist. Since at the outbreak of World War II forced conscription had little real effect on the mountain people, one young Georgian general decided to go personally to try to recruit Svan fighters. The people answered his urgent plea by saying that Hitler had not made them angry and that they would not fight with him. As the German forces invaded the Northern Caucasus, the war began to affect even the isolated Svans. A German shell fell on a Svan village, destroying a house and wounding some people. Only then did the Svans send a message to the Soviet army that now they were angry and ready to fight.

As the Germans penetrated the mountains, the Svans proved highly useful. Once, for example, German snipers established a well-protected nest overlooking an important mountain pass and prevented the advance of troops. The young Georgian general came again to the Svans to ask if there were any mountain people who could approach the nest from above, through the mountains, and kill the snipers. Yes, there were several Svans, in hiding in the woods because of a blood feud, who might undertake this task for him. They agreed to meet with the general only when he promised to come unarmed. At the meeting, they agreed to kill the snipers if the general, in turn, would try to get them amnesty from the Soviet government and try to reconcile the two feuding families. The general gave his word, and, shortly thereafter, the men returned, having killed the snipers.

Promises, pledges, and oral agreements are taken very seriously in cultures without writing. The general was able to keep his word and get amnesty for the men. Reconciling the two families was somewhat more difficult, however, since the blood feud had been going on for several generations and its cause had long been forgotten. The feud was finally resolved by firing a cannon symbolically in the direction of the enemy family. Each member of the injured clan participated in loading the cannon by contributing a bit of gun powder. The score was evened and the blood feud terminated.

9
LIFE'S RHYTHM: CONCLUSIONS ABOUT LONGEVITY

Four years of intensive research and field work among the long-living people of the Caucasus have given me some insights. I met with many physicians in the local academies and gerontological institutes and examined their records on the centenarians. In addition, the notes of my fellow ethnographers studying the Caucasians, and above all the long-lived themselves who spoke freely of their lives and their families, have led me to some conclusions and allowed me to elucidate the major factors which promote their good health and longevity.

CONTINUITY

A rhythmic regularity characterizes Caucasian life and is probably a major source of its healthfulness. Order in daily routines and in the entire arc of life from cradle to grave contributes to the security of the individual and the group. Continuity and regulation in diet, work, sex life, and leisure appear to lessen the strain on the body by avoiding sudden discontinuities and changes.

The days of discomfort experienced by someone who makes a long airplane trip across time zones—jet lag—may provide clues about the causes of psychiatric and somatic illnesses.

Experiments by Dr. Charles Stroebel at the Institute of Living in Hartford show that rhythmicity has a definite relationship to mental health. Monkeys deprived of their regular schedules and subjected to chaotic living develop psychosomatic disorders such as ulcers.

In the Caucasus, life moves at a sure and steady pace and the regular routines are rarely violated. There are no abrupt changes to disrupt the order of their lives, an order established and perpetuated through many generations. This evenness of pace is conducive to serenity, makes for a good general mood, gives a feeling of well-being, and encourages longevity.

CONTINUITY IN WORK PATTERNS

In the Ukraine, Lithuania, Moldavia, Byelorussia, and Abkhasia continuity of occupation is typical of the long-lived. Research by E.I. Stezhenskaya indicates that 80.6 per cent of the longevous people in these republics are pastoral and agricultural workers; 91.4 per cent never changed their occupation and over 60 per cent continued to work after seventy years of age.

CONTINUITY IN DIET

According to data collected by B.S. Martson on the same populations, longevous people had not changed their food habits during their entire lives. The majority are very moderate in their food intake and have lean bodies.

Children, adults, and old people all consume the same diet and seem to have no interest in trying new foods. It is not a matter of having no alternatives, or being confined to locally grown foods; they truly love their traditional foods and see no reason for change or variety.

HEALTH CARE

Longevous persons have a great desire to be healthy and strong. They believe that cleanliness and regular sleeping and eating habits contribute to longevity. Prophylactic and therapeutic herbs, in which they place great faith, are important in their health care. It is interesting that not one of the long-living individuals I interviewed, regardless of religious background, attributed his or her longevity to Providence. Invariably they replied that it was "the good life," which means order, restraint, physical work, and care of one's health. This was true for all ethnic groups.

Pavlov's view was that early aging is caused by constant overtaxing of the nervous system.

REALISTIC LIFE GOALS

Clearly defined behavior patterns and achievable life goals reduce emotional tensions. The Caucasians live in a stable culture where expectations do not overreach the possibilities of attainment and where competition, if found at all, is in nonvital activities such as sports, dancing, and music.

ROLE OF AGED IN COMMUNITY AND FAMILY

In the Caucasus, old people continue to be included in the active life of the kin group and the community. The kinship system promotes longevity by providing a large network of relatives with mutual rights and obligations. There is no cut-off point at a certain age. In all the record books of the collectives, the *oldest* person is listed as the head of the household, regardless of his or her actual contribution or achievement. Khfaf Lazuria, for instance, an uneducated woman of 139, was listed as head of her household. Old people continue to vote, make decisions, and participate in all the activities of which they are capable until death.

After examining the records of 15,000 old people from Georgia and Abkhasia, Pitskhelauri concluded that only married people live to a very old age. Botkin and Kadjan's data also indicate that married people are more likely to reach the age of seventy than are single people. Women who have had children are likewise more likely to reach old age than are those who have remained childless.

The aged, surrounded by numerous respectful progeny of several generations, retain a feeling of individual worth and importance that prolongs useful life. Participating fully in family and community life and retaining a positive self-image reduce the physical and mental problems of aging.

The poet Gamzatov, himself a Caucasian, once questioned an old woman who knew hundreds of curses. He asked her which was the most terrifying she could think of. Her answer illuminates some of the Caucasian values which are conducive to long life. The worst curse she could imagine, she said, was this: "Let there be no old folk in your house to give you wise counsel, and no young people to heed their advice."

EXERCISE

Many Soviet physicians believe that regular exercise, such as walking up and down slopes in mountainous regions, helps develop resistance to diseases and consequently is a factor in longevity. But a comparison with the Hutzuls of the Carpathian mountains, where I did some field work years ago, indicates that such physical factors alone cannot account for longevity. Social and cultural factors appear to be of even greater importance. Hutzul society is youth-oriented and small families predominate; older individuals are not in the same privileged position as in the Caucasus and there are not as many of them.

The attitude toward the old in the Caucasian Nart epics reflects a curious ambivalence, in view of the reverence and homage afforded to old people in the life of the society. It may well be that in the legends, an unconscious resentment of the prevailing rigid patriarchal system finds an acceptable outlet; these feelings could never be expressed overtly.

In the epics old people are, of course, treated as wise and deserving of respect, but not without qualification. From an Ossetinian narrative we learn that in the hunt, the first shots belong to the elderly, after which the younger men may shoot. In the division of the catch, the old men have the unquestioned right to claim the better part. During war marches, the young warriors had to carry and prepare food, feed the older warriors, help them disrobe for the night, and see to it that they had a comfortable place to sleep.

However, the old were deprived of the reverence accorded to them whenever loss of physical strength prevented them from participating in war or the hunt. There are even some terrifying stories of old men being thrown into an abyss to end their useless lives.

There are many variants of narratives concerning the killing of men who were very old and useless. (It is interesting to note that old women are not threatened with death. This may reflect the powerlessness of women and, perhaps, provide further evidence of an unconscious resentment against the patriarchy.) A Kabardinian epic contains the following plot: When Badynoko was born, his parents were already quite old. At the time, the Narts observed a dreadful custom. An old person was considered decrepit and useless when he was no longer able to mount a horse without help, or draw his sword instantly from the sheath, or shoot an arrow at a flying bird, or watch over sheep in the pasture without falling asleep. When no longer able to perform these feats, an old person was set in a basket, taken to a high peak called the "Mountain of Old Age," and flung into the abyss.

When Badynoko grew up, his father was already a decrepit old man. Badynoko loved his father and could not bear to see him killed in this way, even though breaking the custom was considered shameful and punishable. He hid his father in a cave and secretly carried food to him.

Hard times befell the Narts. An unknown disease killed many sheep, crops failed, and hunger threatened the people. Badynoko went to his father for counsel; he repeated what the old man told him to his fellow Narts. The advice was always good and useful, and the Narts praised Badynoko and were grateful to him. He then revealed the truth. It was his father, said Badynoko, and not he who had imparted to them the experience and wisdom which had helped them survive.

The Narts held a council and decided that killing old people is foolish as well as cruel. They decided to honor old people and to listen to their advice in the future. Badynoko's father said, "I cannot work or fight any longer, but I can think."

SELF-IMAGE AND THE EXPECTATION OF LONG LIFE

Social and medical attitudes toward aging are important in the self-image of the elderly. In areas of great longevity, mental and physical deterioration are not viewed as inevitable in old age. The expectation is for a long and useful life, and the old behave in accordance with that expectation. Individuals brought up in areas of high longevity expect to live far beyond the age of one hundred. When old persons are asked to what age they expect to live, they do not care to speculate and thus set limits. A young person will usually answer, "I will live very long, even longer than my great-grandfather."

In the U.S., young adults feel negative about aging. Older Americans feel a deepening resentment about "forced retirement."

In 1971, an article of mine on old age in Abkhasia was published in *The New York Times Magazine*. The response amazed me. The majority of non-professionals who took the time to write were older people, mostly women. Anxiety and wistfulness shone through these letters. The writers longed for a solution to their problems, and envied the Abkhasians—for one cannot make up for years of abusing one's body and emotions. They saw Abkhasia as a Shangri-La—which it is not. Abhkasia is tough, with strict rules. Most Westerners would find the unspontaneous, formalistic, and measured way of life constricting. They would miss their cherished freedom, individuality, and creativity.

Placing old people in a special closed milieu is unquestionably tragic, whatever one sees as its justification. The "old people's home" deprives the elderly of their social value and, consequently, of their desire to live.

Isolation and loneliness can kill a human being. In order for human beings to function they must be engaged in meaningful activities and must be involved in meaningful relationships with other human beings. The human organism must receive a whole range of sensations and impressions. If a person is deprived of sensations, of light, sound, touch, and so on, he loses his sense of involvement with others and with the world. As experiments in the space program have shown, a person deprived of the normal everyday impressions begins to lose his sense of reality and his sense of his own identity.

In the Caucasus, the old people remain involved in their family, their lineage, and their community. They are involved emotionally and physically. Their work provides them not only with physical exercise but also with the knowledge of their own meaningful contribution to their community.

It is my feeling that the high incidence of longevity in the Caucasus is a result of the complete immersion of the individual in an atmosphere of inner, consistent values, creating a biological and spiritual rhythm. There is no lost energy spent attempting to introduce elements alien to the established patterns of life into the culture, resulting in a conflict-free, uncompetitive society.

The healthier, happier old age of the Caucasus does not provide us with ready answers for our own society, but it at least points to possible ways to ameliorate the plight of our aged. The subject should command the attention of all of us, for old age is our common fate.

10
SOME RECIPES FROM THE LONG-LIVING PEOPLE OF THE CAUCASUS

Many people have asked me about how the people of the Caucasus eat (indicating, I suppose, our preoccupation with food!). I have in earlier chapters described the diet, its nutritional aspects, and its general content. But here I thought it would be especially interesting and fun to present readers with some good (and tested!) recipes from genuine, and delicious, Caucasian meals. Since I have come home, I have prepared these very dishes for friends and colleagues and have been successful, I think, in showing them how tasty as well as healthful the dishes are.

Food is always, of course, the most conservative item to put in, or take out, of a culture. In the Caucasus, where Western dress and other Western forms have become accepted, food, other than Caucasian, is still considered second-rate, neither tasty nor worthwhile to eat. Those who have gone to the cities and must make do with some substitutes can't wait to go home and eat their natural rural meals, and many packages are sent to the urban areas by understanding relatives.

The recipes that follow are from various regions. Whenever I ate something I really loved, I stopped and took down the recipe. Only a few had to be adapted because of special spices.

In the recipes, I often mention spices without listing a measurement. The Caucasians use a great deal of spice, especially in their sauces, and some Americans may find it too sharp. It took me some time to get used to eating Caucasian foods. Therefore I leave the particular amounts up to the individual. The food will not diminish in taste with a lessening of spice.

SOUPS

Khash Soup   Georgia

2 lbs. beef or mutton feet	Sauce: Salt
1 lb. soup bones	3 cloves garlic, minced
Water	1 tsp. radish
Milk	½ cup bouillon

In Georgia there are several other variants. For this recipe, carefully clean and scrape the feet and bones, cut them into pieces, and place them into a pot of boiling water to cover well. When the water returns to a boil, pour the water off, and pour more boiling water over the meat. Cook the meat slowly until it begins to come off the bone, constantly removing the foam and fat. Then place the bones in a separate dish; pour in enough milk to cover the bones; cover the dish and allow it to stand for five or six hours. Pour out the milk, and transfer the feet and bones to a clean pot, and brown them over a low flame for fifteen minutes. Pour off the juice which forms into a pot, and allow the meat to stew for another 30 to 40 minutes, constantly pouring the juice off. Then pour boiling water and the juice into the pot with the bones and simmer another five or six hours.

Mix the ingredients for the sauce together. Serve the sauce separately, and add to *Khash* as desired.

Khash Soup   Armenia

2 lbs. beef or mutton feet	Sauce: Salt
1 lb. soup bones	3 cloves garlic, minced
Water	1 tsp. radish
	½ cup bouillon

Carefully clean and scrape the feet and bones. Cut them into pieces, and wash them in cold water. Immerse the meat in water so that it is covered by several inches. *Khash* is cooked without salt. Cook until the bouillon becomes thick and the meat separates easily from the bones. Frequently discard the brown foam that forms on the surface along with the excess fat. *Khash* is served very hot.

Mix the ingredients for the sauce together. It is served separately, added to *Khash* as desired. This method of preparing *Khash* is widespread in Armenia, where the dish is eaten in the morning for breakfast.

Chikhirtma Soup   Georgia

3 large onions, finely chopped	½ tsp. cinnamon	Juice of 1 lemon
1 tbsp. vegetable oil or margarine	¼ tsp. coriander	1 egg
1 tbsp. flour or corn starch	Pepper	Parsley
4 cups chicken broth	Wine vinegar	

Slice the onion into sections and chop finely. Sauté the onion in the vegetable oil while sprinkling in the flour. Bring the chicken broth to a boil and add the sautéed onions. Add the cinnamon, coriander, pepper, and wine vinegar. Allow to cook over a low flame for 10 minutes. Add the lemon juice, stir, and turn off the flame. Then add a well-beaten egg, stirring constantly. Sprinkle with parsley.

Bozbash Soup   Azerbaijan

1 lb. lamb	½ lb. string beans	Salt
Water	2 eggplants	Pepper
4 onions, finely chopped	3 green peppers	Parsley
10 potatoes	Vegetable oil	Dill
8 tomatoes	1½ tbsp. tomato purée	

Wash the lamb in cold water. Cut it into small pieces. Place in saucepan. Cover with water and bring to a boil on a low flame. Add finely chopped onion and cook 40 minutes on a slow flame. Fifteen minutes before the soup has finished cooking, add potatoes (cut in half if large).

Cut up and brown fresh tomatoes, string beans, eggplant, and green peppers in a frying pan in oil; then add the tomato purée. Add these ingredients to the soup. Salt and pepper the soup and bring it to a boil. Before serving sprinkle with parsley and dill.

Kharcho Soup   Georgia

1 lb. shoulder or neck lamb	Salt
Water	Pepper
2 onions, finely chopped	4 tbsp. tomato purée or
2–3 cloves garlic, finely chopped	2–3 fresh tomatoes, skinned
½ cup rice	Parsley
½ cup marinated plums	Dill

Cut the meat into little pieces with bones, calculating 3 to 4 pieces per portion. Cover with cold water and boil, periodically removing the foam that forms on the surface. After 1½ hours, place the finely chopped onion and garlic in the pot, along with the rice, marinated plums, salt, and pepper, and cook for another 30 minutes.

Fry the tomato purée or the skinned fresh tomatoes separately for 5 to 10 minutes and add to the soup. Before serving, sprinkle the soup with finely chopped parsley and dill.

Chikhirtma Soup Made from Chicken or Lamb   Georgia

5 onions, finely chopped	Salt
Fat from chicken or lamb	¼ tsp. cinnamon
1 whole chicken or 2 lbs. lamb	Freshly ground black pepper
Water	2–3 eggs
4 sprigs coriander	1–2 tbsp. wine vinegar

Chop or grind up onions finely. Brown lightly in a frying pan in mutton or chicken fat. Then place the chicken or lamb, cut up into small pieces, into the pan and allow the mixture to cook for 10 to 15 minutes. Transfer the mixture to a pot and pour cold water (8 to 10 cups) over the meat and onions, Boil for 2 to 2½ hours. Ten minutes before the soup is finished boiling, add finely chopped coriander, salt, and ground cinnamon. Black pepper may also be added.

Before serving, beat 2 to 3 eggs with the wine vinegar, and add to the soup, stirring constantly. Then bring the soup to a boil and remove from the flame. Serves four.

Noodles with Nuts Soup   Georgia

1 lb. walnuts, shelled and chopped	1 lb. prepared noodles
Water	1 clove garlic, minced (optional)
3 onions, finely chopped	

Place the chopped shelled walnuts in a saucepan. Cover with 6 cups of cold water. Bring it to a boil and add onions. Now add the prepared noodles and allow to boil until the dough becomes soft. Minced garlic can be added to the soup.

Chikhirtma Soup Made from Chicken   Georgia

1 chicken, 3–3½ lb.	Black pepper
Water	Coriander seeds
Salt	Wine vinegar to taste
1 lb. onions, chopped	3–4 eggs
1 tbsp. flour	Juice of 1 lemon
3–4 sprigs coriander	Saffron
Cinnamon	3–4 sprigs parsley, finely chopped

Place the chicken in a saucepan and cover with 8 to 10 cups cold water. Cover and allow to cook for 1 to 2 hours, removing the foam that forms on the surface with a skimmer. Take the chicken out of the bouillon, place it on a plate, and salt to taste. Skim the fat from the surface of the bouillon. Place the fat in a clean pot, add chopped onions, and brown them. Pour a tablespoon of flour, dissolved in a cup of bouillon, over the sautéed onions. Then add 7 to 8 cups of chicken bouillon and bring the broth to a boil. Add the coriander greens. After 30 minutes, add the cinnamon, black pepper, ground coriander seeds, wine vinegar and salt (to taste). Continue boiling for 15 minutes. Remove the soup from the stove, remove the coriander greens, and add the eggs while stirring. Then return the soup to the stove and bring it to a boil. Quickly remove the soup from the stove—do not allow it to boil. Add lemon juice and a pinch of saffron.

When serving, place pieces of chicken in the soup and sprinkle with finely chopped parsley. The soup can also be served without the chicken; in this case the chicken can be used as a second course.

MEAT DISHES

Shashlyk   (Shishkebab)   Azerbaijan

1½ lbs. lamb or mutton	1 oz. butter or margarine
Salt	4–5 scallions
Pepper	4 fresh tomatoes
2 onions, finely chopped	3–4 tbsp. *tkemali* sauce (see *Sauces*)
Parsley	12–16 dried or fresh barberries (or 1 lemon)
5 tbsp. lemon juice	Dill

Cube mutton, place in china or enameled pot with salt, pepper, finely chopped onions, parsley, lemon juice; cover and marinate in refrigerator 4 to 5 hours. Marinate lamb *without* vinegar. Skewer meat, rub with butter or margarine and roast over hot wood coals without flames, turning constantly. Serve with coarsely cut scallions, parsley, dill, tomatoes, slices of lemon, *tkemali* sauce, and barberry. Serves four.

Chicken-Tabaka   Georgia

4 spring chickens	Lettuce
8 cloves garlic, chopped	4 fresh tomatoes
Salt	Scallions
Pepper	1 large or 2 medium onions
5 tbsp. clarified butter	10–12 tbsp. *tkemali* or garlic sauce (see *Sauces*)

Cut chickens lengthwise, spread open, dry, and rub with chopped garlic, salt, and pepper. Place in hot frying pan with clarified butter, spread open, and cover with weighted lid. Fry for 20 to 30 minutes over medium flame until crusty. Turn and brown the other side.

Before serving, decorate with small pieces of lettuce. Serve tomatoes, scallions, onions cut into slices and sauce separately. Serves four.

Cutlets   Armenia

1 lb. boneless beef cutlets	Salt
2 large onions	Pepper
½ lb. goat cheese	½ cup milk
Flour	Bread crumbs
2 eggs	Vegetable oil for deep frying
	Melted butter

Press cutlets into thin patties without tearing. Chop and sauté onion and add it to the cheese. Fold a portion of the cheese into each cutlet, forming a little pyramid. Powder with flour; coat with eggs beaten with salt, pepper, and milk; cover with bread crumbs. Allow to stand for 10 to 15 minutes in the refrigerator. Fry 5 to 6 min. in deep fat hot enough to smoke. Serve two cutlets per person with melted butter and french-fried potatoes, which can be cooked in the same oil. Serves four.

Cerkes Tavugu (Circassian chicken)   Circassia

1 chicken, 5 lbs.	1 teaspoon salt
Water	Pepper
1 large onion, quartered	2 cups walnuts
1 carrot	1 tbsp. paprika
1 bunch parsley	3 slices white bread

Place chicken in saucepan and cover with water. Add onion, carrot, parsley, salt, and pepper. Bring to a boil and skim off foam on top. Cover and cook until chicken is tender. Remove from pot and allow to cool. Save stock. When cool, remove skin and bones, and cut chicken into small pieces. Put walnuts through meat grinder twice. Save red walnut oil for garnish.* Add paprika. Soak bread in chicken stock. Squeeze it dry and add it to walnuts and paprika. Mix well. Run bread-paprika-walnut mixture through grinder three times. Add 1 cup of chicken stock. Work into a paste. Divide the paste in half. Use half to coat pieces of chicken. Arrange chicken in bowl, and spread the other half of the paste over it. Sprinkle with additional paprika and drops of walnut oil. Serve cold.

Satsivi   Georgia

1 turkey, 10 lbs. or less	Paprika (to taste)
Water	2 tsp. coriander, ground
1 lb. walnuts, chopped	¼ tsp. ginger, ground
2 cloves garlic, minced	1 lb. onions, chopped
Salt	½ c. wine vinegar

Wash and boil the turkey, half-immersed in water for 30 minutes. Bring to a boil and skim off foam on top. Cover and cook until about half done. Remove from pan and allow it to cool. Set the broth aside. Roast the turkey until done. Cool. *Satsivi* means cooled in Georgian.

Mix the walnuts, garlic, salt, and paprika. Mix coriander and ginger with a little of the broth. Cook half the onions in the broth. Then add the spices and onions to the rest of the turkey broth along with the wine vinegar to make a sauce. Cool. Then cut the turkey into pieces and place on a serving dish.

*Walnuts bought in cans or packages are usually dried; oil will not form. You can buy walnut oil in health-food stores.

Sprinkle with the remaining chopped onions and pour the cool sauce over it. *Satsivi* is usually served with rice.

Fisidzhan Pilaf   Azerbaijan

¼ lb. rice	1 cup Bouillon
½ lb. shoulder or neck lamb (for stew)	1 small onion, chopped
Salt	½ cup walnuts, chopped
5 tbsp. clarified butter	½ cup pomegranate kernels
	Cinnamon

Prepare boiled rice separately in the usual manner. Cut the lamb into pieces, add salt, and brown it in butter in a hot frying pan. (Chopped lamb or chicken can be substituted for stewing lamb. If chopped lamb is used, make small patties or meatballs.) Gradually add a cup of bouillon, the chopped onions and walnuts, pomegranate kernels, and cinnamon to the frying pan, and allow it to cook on a low flame. The rice is served in small mounds on warmed plates. The *fisidzhan* can be served separately or on the side of the plate.

Chicken in Walnut Sauce (A Banquet Dish)   Abkhasia
(A variation of *Satsivi,* a Georgian dish)

1 chicken, 2–3½ lbs.	1 cup onions, chopped
Salt	2 cloves garlic, crushed
1 tsp. saffron threads	1 tbsp. flour, sifted
Water	¼ tsp. coriander
3 cups good stock or bouillon	1 tsp. red pepper, ground
3 lbs. shelled walnuts	1 tsp. fresh dill, chopped
½ cup wine vinegar	3 hard-boiled eggs
⅛ lb. butter or margarine (½ stick)	(mash yolks and shred whites)
	2 sprigs fresh parsley, chopped

Chicken

Wash and dry the chicken. Sprinkle with salt. Roast, sealed in aluminum foil to keep moist and to prevent overbrowning. Do not cover pan; do not add water. Cook at 325° F for 1½ hours. When done, cool and cut into serving portions.

Sauce

Dissolve saffron in 2 tablespoons boiling water and add to bouillon. Set aside. Chop shelled walnuts coarsely and place them in a bowl. Bring vinegar to a boil and pour over walnuts. Let stand.

Melt butter in a saucepan. Add chopped onions and crushed garlic. Cook until onions are transparent but not browned. Sprinkle with sifted flour. Gradually add one cup of bouillon, stirring frequently. Add coriander, ground red pepper, dill, mashed egg yolks, and salt to taste. Add the second cup of bouillon and bring to a boil. Turn off heat. Add walnut mixture and mix well.

Place chicken parts in a serving dish, cover with the prepared sauce and refrigerate overnight. This dish can be prepared two or three days in advance. Before serving, gently stir in the reserved third cup of bouillon to make the sauce more liquid. Sprinkle with chopped parsley and whites of eggs (optional).

The Abkhasians often boil the chicken in a small amount of water instead of roasting it; if they use this procedure, they add a bay leaf, one or two quartered onions, soup greens, a few peppercorns, and two minced cloves of garlic. The stock is then used for the sauce.

Chygyrtma Pilaf   Azerbaijan

1 chicken, 2½–3 lbs.	Juice of ½ lemon
Salt	Cinnamon
1/3 cup butter	2 eggs
2 medium onions, chopped	Dill (optional)
	½ lb. rice

Wash the chicken and cut it into serving pieces. Salt and brown it in butter in a hot frying pan. Add onions, lemon juice, and cinnamon. Pour well-beaten eggs over the chicken. Dill is sometimes added to the eggs. Transfer this mixture to a baking dish and cook in a 350°F oven until ready. Boil the rice and serve it separately.

Raisin and Honey Chicken   Georgia

1 chicken, 2½–3 lbs.	Water
Salt	⅛ lb. margarine or butter (½ stick)
Lemon (optional)	2 tbsp. honey
½ cup seedless raisins	½ cup uncooked rice

Wash the chicken in salted water and dry. (Optional: The chicken can be rubbed with lemon inside and outside.) Boil the raisins for five minutes in just enough water to cover them. Drain and transfer into small frying pan. Sauté raisins with butter and honey. Add this mixture to the uncooked rice, mixing thoroughly. Place stuffing in the cavity of the chicken, closing the cavity with skewers. Bake in open pan at 350° F until done.

Chicken Kish-Mish   Azerbaijan

1 chicken, 2½–3 lbs.	½ cup seedless raisins
Salt	½ cup walnuts, chopped
Water	1 medium onion, chopped
	⅛ lb. margarine or butter (½ stick)

This dish, whose title literally means "raisins," is a variant of the Georgian Raisin and Honey Chicken. Prepare the chicken in the same manner, but prepare the stuffing somewhat differently. Sautée the raisins, chopped walnuts, and onion together in the butter, mix, and place in cavity of the chicken. Close the cavity with skewers, and bake in an open pan at 350° F until done.

Sendzhan Pilaf   Azerbaijan

1 lb. lamb	Pepper
½ cup walnuts	Cooking oil
Salt	Vinegar

Grind up the meat and walnuts in a meat grinder and mix in a bowl with salt and pepper. Shape the mixture into patties and cook in oil. Vinegar is used as a sauce.

Serve with rice.

Cherkessian Pilaf   Cherkessia

1 cup rice	1 tsp. butter
Water	½ cup raisins
Salt	2 tbsp. honey

Cook the rice in water with a dash of salt and a teaspoon of butter. Add raisins and honey five minutes before the rice is ready. Serve with yogurt.

Lamb with Apples   Armenia

1½ lbs. lamb	6 cooking apples	Salt
Water	1 red pepper	Sugar
¼ lb. margarine or butter (1 stick)	1 carrot	Parsley
2 large onions, finely chopped		

Cut lamb into pieces and boil in enough water to cover until half cooked. Strain off the bouillon and reserve it. Brown the lamb in butter or margarine in a saucepan. Add bouillon to just cover the meat. Cover and stew until the meat is almost done. Add finely chopped sautéed onions, apples, cored and cut into sections, chopped red pepper, and grated carrot. Add salt and sugar to taste. Allow the lamb to continue to stew on the top of the stove or in the oven until ready. Sprinkle with parsley. Serves four.

Chakhokhbili   Georgia

1 spring chicken	2 tbsp. vegetable oil	2–3 sprigs fresh basil
Salt	Black or hot pepper	1½ lbs. tomatoes
3–4 onions, minced	4–5 sprigs fresh coriander	

Wash the chicken and cut it into small pieces. Add salt. Place it in a deep frying pan or saucepan with minced onions. Add oil and stew over a low flame until the onion browns. Then add the black or hot pepper, coriander sprigs, and basil (both finely chopped), and sectioned tomatoes. Cover the pot and slowly cook until chicken is done. Serves four.

Cherkessian Lamb Stew

1 lb. lamb (stewing meat)	2 medium onions
1 tbsp. butter or margarine	1 tbsp. flour
	½ cup water

Cube the lamb and fry in butter in a frying pan with the chopped onions. After the meat is browned, add the flour, mixed with water, and stew over a low flame until done. Usually served over noodles.

Turshi Kaurma Pilaf   Azerbaijan

1½ lbs. lamb	Cinnamon	Salt
5 tbsp. clarified butter	Saffron	½ cup chestnuts
½ cup bouillon	Pepper	2 oz. sorrel
Cloves		

Cut the lamb into pieces and brown in a frying pan with butter. Add the bouillon along with the spices, chestnuts, and sorrel. Cover the pan and cook over a low flame until ready. Baked eggplants make an excellent garnish. Serve rice separately.

FISH DISHES

Steamed Fish with Tomatoes   Georgia

1 lb. fish fillet	3 sprigs fresh coriander
Salt	Water
3 onions, chopped	1 lb. fresh tomatoes
	Hot peppers

Cut fish into portions; place in pan; sprinkle with salt, chopped onions, and coriander; half cover with water; cover and place over low flame. Boil tomatoes one minute, skin, and sauté. Place cooked fish in bowls, add tomatoes, salt, and chopped hot peppers.

Fish in Pomegranate Sauce   Georgia

1 lb. fish	1–2 tbsp. vegetable oil
Salt	Hot peppers
1–2 tbsp. wheat or corn flour	1½ cups pomegranate juice
	Pomegranate seeds

Cut fish into portions. Boil in lightly salted water until half-cooked. Coat with flour, fry in oil on both sides until crusty. To serve, add chopped hot pepper to pomegranate juice, and pour over fish. Sprinkle with pomegranate seeds and serve.

Swordfish Stewed with Vegetables   All Caucasia

1–2 carrots	Salt
2 onions	5 black peppercorns
1½ lbs. swordfish	1–2 laurel leaves
1 cup water	½ cup cream
	1 tbsp. sweet butter

Combine cut carrots, onions, and fish in cooking pot. Add hot water, salt, and seasonings. Cover and cook 30 minutes over low flame. Serve with sauce of warmed cream and melted sweet butter.

Boiled potatoes and cauliflower make excellent garnishes.

Swordfish Baked with Eggs   All Caucasia

1½ lbs. boiled swordfish	4 tbsp. vegetable oil
Salt	2 eggs
Black pepper	1½ cups milk
1–2 tbsp. breadcrumbs	1 tbsp. grated cheese

Cut fish into small pieces. Season with salt and pepper, cover with breadcrumbs, sauté briefly in oil. Combine eggs and milk and pour the mixture over the fish. Sprinkle with grated cheese and breadcrumbs, and bake.

Whipped potatoes or stewed vegetables are the best garnishes.

VEGETABLE DISHES

Pilaf (Rice)   All Caucasia

2 cups uncooked rice	⅛ lb. butter (½ stick)
4 medium tomatoes,	3½ cups water, meat stock, or chicken
peeled, seeded, and cubed	broth
	2 tsp. salt

Wash and drain rice well. Place tomatoes and butter in a pan and simmer until tomato paste forms. Add liquid and salt and boil for 2 minutes. Add rice while liquid is boiling. Stir once, cover, and cook over medium heat without stirring until rice has absorbed all liquid. Turn flame low and simmer for 20 minutes. Keep covered after removing from fire.

Purée of Red Kidney Beans with Cornelian Cherries   Abkhasia

1 lb. red kidney beans	3 oz. almonds
Water	2 oz. seedless raisins
Salt	4 oz. cornelian cherries

Soak the kidney beans overnight. Cook with a small amount of water for several hours until ready. Salt after the beans are completely cooked. Strain the beans, reserving the broth. Mash the beans well with a wooden spoon.

Scald the almonds with boiling water, skin and cut them into slivers. Wash the raisins and dried cornelian cherries. Soak them for 15 to 20 minutes. Place

177

the mashed red kidney beans in a frying pan with the cherries, almonds, and raisins. Salt and add ½ cup of the broth in which the kidney beans were cooked. Cook over a slow flame for 20 to 25 minutes, mixing periodically. Serve.

Lobio (Kidney Beans)   Abkhasia

2–3 cups red kidney beans	5 cloves garlic, finely chopped
Water	Coriander
Salt	Dill
Freshly ground black pepper	2 onions, chopped
	1 lb. shelled walnuts, chopped

Soak the kidney beans overnight. Cook with a small amount of water for several hours until ready. Salt after the beans are completely cooked. Mash well with a wooden spoon. Add the pepper, garlic, and spices to taste. Sauté the chopped onions and mix in with the beans. Add chopped walnuts. Allow to cool before eating. *Lobio* is often eaten for breakfast. For the Abkhasians, it is a ritual dish made for every important occasion.

Stewed Mushrooms with Nuts   Georgia

1 lb. mushrooms	½ clove garlic
2 tbsp. vegetable oil	4 sprigs coriander
Salt	¼ cup wine vinegar
½ cup walnuts	4 sprigs dill

Clean and dice mushrooms. Place in a saucepan with vegetable oil and salt, and stew for 1 hour.

Chop up the walnuts with the garlic, salt, coriander. Add the wine vinegar. Add this mixture to the mushrooms, mix, and cook on a slow flame for five minutes. Before serving, sprinkle with dill.

Beans with Wine Vinegar and Vegetable Oil   Georgia

1 lb. string beans	3 onions, chopped
Water	1/3 cup vegetable oil
Salt	Freshly ground black pepper
	½ cup wine vinegar

Boil the beans in salted water until tender and drain the water; reserve ¼ cup. Brown the onions in the vegetable oil. Add salt, black pepper, wine vinegar, and mix. Sauté for another 2 to 3 minutes. Then add this mixture to the beans, adding the water in which the beans were cooked. Allow to cook for 1 to 2 minutes, drain, and serve.

Eggplant with Nuts   Azerbaijan

2 lbs. eggplant	½ cup basil
1 cup water	¾ cup parsley
1 cup walnuts	¾ cup celery
2 cloves garlic	½ cup savory
Salt	2 onions, chopped
Hot pepper	Wine vinegar or pomegranate juice
½ cup coriander greens,	Cinnamon (optional)
finely chopped	Cloves (optional)

Cut eggplants lengthwise and place in a frying pan; add 1 cup of boiling water and cook 20 to 30 minutes. Strain the eggplants well and strip off the skin. Chop the walnuts, garlic, and salt together or grind them in a meat grinder. Mix this thoroughly with the hot pepper, herbs, chopped onions, and wine vinegar or pomegranate juice (you may also add cinnamon and cloves). Either pour this sauce over the eggplants in a dish or mix it with the eggplant. Cook the mixture for an hour in a saucepan to remove the bitterness.

Sometimes, eggplant cooked in vegetable oil is used. In this case, cook the eggplants until half ready; squeeze out excess water and brown the vegetable lightly on all sides. Use the same nut sauce. Before serving, sprinkle with chopped parsley and pomegranate seeds.

Eggplant with Nuts is also eaten in Georgia for breakfast or as an appetizer before lunch and supper, but it is served cold.

String Beans with Nuts and Vinegar   Georgia

¾ lb. string beans	Wine vinegar (or pomegranate juice
Water	or damson plum sauce)
Salt	2–3 onions or scallions
½–1 cup walnuts	3–4 sprigs basil
1–2 cloves garlic	Parsley
Hot peppers	Dill
Coriander	Pomegranate seeds

Cut up the beans, cook in salted water until tender, and strain in a colander. Allow to cool and press out excess water. Grind up the walnuts, salt, garlic, hot peppers, and coriander. Add wine vinegar (pomegranate juice or damson plum sauce can substituted), chopped onions or scallions, basil, parsley, dill. Mix all with the string beans. Sprinkle the beans with parsley or pomegranate seeds and serve.

String Beans with Buttermilk   Georgia

1 lb. string beans	Parsley
Water	2–3 sprigs mint
Salt	Coriander
2 cups buttermilk	Hot pepper
3 sprigs basil	3–4 cloves garlic

Cut up the string beans, boil in salted water until tender, and strain through a colander. Allow to cool, and press out excess water. Beat the buttermilk well, and pour it over the string beans; then mix in the finely cut basil, parsley, mint, coriander, salt, hot pepper, and garlic.

Beans with Nuts and Wine Vinegar   Georgia

1 lb. string beans	1 clove garlic
Water	Hot pepper
Salt	½–1 cup wine vinegar
½ cup walnuts	2 onions, chopped
4 sprigs coriander	2 leeks, finely chopped
	2 sprigs parsley

Cook the beans in salted water until tender. Drain, reserving ¼ cup water. Grind up the walnuts, coriander, garlic, hot pepper, and salt. Mix with vinegar and add chopped onions, finely chopped leeks, and chopped parsley. Mix with the cooked beans, add reserved water, and cook for another 10 to 15 minutes. Then cool.

Spring Salad   Georgia

4 tomatoes	Sugar to taste
2 cucumbers	½ cup wine vinegar
½ lb. lettuce	1 cup shredded cabbage
¾ lb. lima beans	1 tsp. chopped dill
2–3 eggs (hard-boiled)	Pepper
Salt to taste	Scallions

Wash the tomatoes and skin and cut the cucumbers into slices. Wash and tear up the lettuce. Cook the lima beans in just enough salt water to cover them; drain and allow to cool. Chop up and salt the hard-boiled eggs. Mix the salt and sugar with the wine vinegar to prepare a dressing. Place the lettuce, lima beans, and cabbage in a salad bowl and dress with wine vinegar. Sprinkle with dill. Place slices of tomatoes and cucumbers over the beans, add salt and pepper. Sprinkle with chopped scallions and the chopped eggs.

Eggplant Salad   Georgia

1 large eggplant (1 lb.)   3 green peppers, seeded and minced
1 clove garlic, minced

Bake eggplant until soft. Remove from oven and take off the dark skin. Chop up the eggplant, using only with wooden or glass utensils. Add the minced garlic and chopped green peppers. Serve cold.

Quince Fruit Salad   Armenia

1 lb. quince   1 cup sugar
Water

Remove the skin from the quince. Cut the fruit in half and place in a saucepan, covering with approximately twice as much water as fruit. Cook with sugar until the quince becomes soft. Serve cold.

String Beans with Eggs   Armenia

1 lb. string beans   Pepper
1 cup diced onions   Sprig parsley, minced
1 tsp. butter   4–5 walnuts, cut
Salt   into small pieces
                          2 eggs

Preheat the oven to 350° F. Trim and wash the beans. Cut them lengthwise. Braise the onions and string beans in butter over a low flame. Sprinkle with salt, pepper, and minced parsley. Place this mixture in a buttered baking dish. Add walnuts. Beat the eggs and pour over the mixture. Bake for 30 minutes or until the beans are done.

Erevan Salad   Armenia

2 large tomatoes	Coriander
2 cucumbers	Basil leaf
1 green pepper	Salt
1 medium onion	Parsley
	Vinegar

Wash tomatoes, cucumbers, green pepper. Skin the cucumbers. Cut out the core and seeds from the green pepper. Peel the onion. Cut the vegetables into round slices. Wash and chop up the coriander leaves, basil leaf, salt, and parsley. Place the vegetables in a salad bowl in layers, alternating the tomatoes, cucumbers, and green pepper. Pour vinegar and sprinkle chopped chives on top.

Armenian Eggplant and Tomato Salad

1 eggplant (1 lb.)	2 medium tomatoes
Salt	1 green pepper
2 tbsp. sunflower seed oil	Pepper
1 large onion	Vinegar
	Parsley

Wash the eggplant, skin and cut it into slices. Salt and allow to it stand for 10 to 15 minutes. Press out the excess water. Brown the eggplant slices in sunflower seed oil with sliced onion. Place in a bowl. Cut tomatoes into thin slices; core and seed green pepper and cut into thin rings. Add salt, pepper, vinegar, and mix. Place in a salad bowl and sprinkle with parsley.

Armenian Eggplant with Cheese

1 eggplant (1 lb.)	1 large green pepper
1 large onion	¼ lb. Parmesan cheese
	4 tbsp. sunflower seed oil

Bake the eggplant. Pour boiling water over the eggplant, skin, and cut into fine pieces. Chop onion. Core, seed, and chop green pepper. Grate cheese finely and mix with vegetables. Add sunflower seed oil. Serve cold.

Arashy: Nut Oil   Abkhasia

¼ tsp. coriander   Salt
¼ tsp. dill   1 cup walnuts
Freshly ground black pepper   2–4 tbsp. walnut oil

The nuts are grated on stones in Abkhasia. Here we can use a nut grater. Grind coriander, dill, freshly ground black pepper, and salt. Add to the nuts and grate. Then add walnut oil (available in health-food stores) and mix.

Achapa   Abkhasia

Water   1 tsp. vinegar or pomegranate juice
1 head white cabbage, coarsely   Dill
chopped   Parsley
Salt   Coriander
½ cup walnuts   Garlic
1 tbsp. butter   2 medium onions

Boil the coarsely chopped cabbage with salt. When soft, strain and pour off the extra water. Put all other ingredients through a meat grinder. Mix together and serve.

This same dish is called *Akhulchapa* when served with *Arashy* or nut oil.

Garlic and Tomato Salad   Armenia

1 clove garlic, finely chopped   Salt
2–2½ tbsp. vinegar   Pepper
2 medium tomatoes   Coriander

Mix finely chopped garlic with vinegar and allow to stand for 30 minutes. Cut the tomatoes into sections, place in a salad bowl, add salt and pepper, and cover with the vinegar-garlic mixture. Sprinkle with coriander.

Akhtsan (String Bean Salad)   Armenia

½ lb. string beans   2–3 scallions
Salt   Black pepper
Water   2–3 tbsps. sunflower seed oil
                                 Vinegar

Cut the string beans up finely, place in a pot with salted boiling water, and cook several minutes. Drain in a sieve and cool. Mix the cooked beans with finely chopped scallions, add pepper, sunflower seed oil, and vinegar.

Skewered Eggplant Salad   Armenia

1 eggplant (½ lb.)	Salt
3 tbsp. sunflower seed oil	Pepper
3–4 scallions	Fresh dill
Dill	Parsley
	Scallions

Wash the eggplant, dry lightly, skewer, and brown over hot coals. Skin the eggplant, cut it into small pieces, add sunflower oil, finely chopped scallions, dill, and salt and pepper. Mix and allow to cool. Transfer the eggplant into a salad bowl or plate and decorate with fresh dill or parsley greens and scallions.

Purée of French Kidney Beans with Onion   Armenia

1 lb. kidney beans	4 tbsp. vegetable oil
Salt	2 large onions, finely chopped
Pepper	Coriander

Soak the kidney beans overnight. Cook with a small amount of water for several hours until ready. Salt after the beans are completely cooked. Grind up cooked kidney beans. Transfer to a plate. Add salt, pepper, and vegetable oil. Sauté finely chopped onions. Sprinkle beans with sautéed onion and coriander, and mix well.

String Bean Salad   Georgia

1 lb. string beans	Hot pepper
Water	1 medium onion, chopped
Salt	4 sprigs fresh dill
	2 tsp. wine vinegar

Clean and cut the string beans. Boil in lightly salted water. Strain. Add salt and hot pepper, and chopped onion and mix. Sprinkle finely chopped dill over the string beans, and mix in wine vinegar.

SAUCES

Note: In sauces in which mint is used, dill and coriander should be used generously.

Nut Sauce   Georgia

1 cup walnuts	2–3 sprigs coriander
½ clove garlic	½ cup pomegranate juice
Salt	¾–1 cup water
Hot pepper	Pomegranate seeds
½ tsp. coriander seeds	Nut oil
½ tsp. ground saffron	

Grind up the walnuts, garlic, salt, hot pepper. Add ground coriander seeds, the saffron, and coriander, and mix well. Dilute the mixture with pomegranate sauce and water. Pour the sauce into a bowl, sprinkle with pomegranate seeds. Pour nut oil (from health-food stores) on top.

Fish Sauce Made from Walnuts   Russia—used in the Caucasus

½ lb. shelled walnuts	1 tbsp. salad oil
3 tbsp. water	1 tsp. powdered sugar
1 tsp. salt	1 tbsp. dried, fine breadcrumbs
2 egg yolks (hard-boiled)	1 tbsp. Russian mustard (or French)
	½ cup vinegar

Grind the walnuts, gradually adding water and salt. Mix well. Grate the yolks and add to the salad oil very slowly, mixing constantly. Then add the sugar, breadcrumbs, and mustard. Mix. Add the vinegar and mix again. This sauce is usually served with broiled fish. It is rarely served separately.

Sauce for Poultry   Georgia

2 cups blackberries	Paprika or pepper
1 cup unripe green grapes	1 sprig dill
3 sprigs fresh coriander or	Salt
½ tsp. crushed coriander	Fried onion (optional)
1 clove garlic, crushed	¼ cup pomegranate juice (optional)

Mash the blackberries and grapes with a wooden spoon and put through a sieve. Add the spices. Then add the onion and pomegranate juice, if desired. Heat the sauce until warm and serve.

Satsibeli Sauce   Georgia

2 cups damson plums	¼ tsp. coriander
Water	Hot pepper
	Salt

Cook unripe damson plums in a small amount of water until the pits separate from the fruit. Strain, add coriander, dried red pepper, and salt. *Satsibeli* is a sauce for all kinds of meats.

Sharp Cherkessian Meat Sauce   Cherkessia

1 cup plain yogurt	¼ tsp. coriander seeds
2 cloves garlic, crushed	Hot Peppers
	Salt

Mix the yogurt with the garlic, coriander seeds, chopped dried red peppers, and salt. This sauce is served with internal organ meat, feet, and head meat.

Garlic Sauce   Georgia

A. 8 cloves garlic	½ tsp. coriander seeds
Salt	¼ cup wine vinegar
	½–¾ cup water

Grind up the garlic in a mortar or use a garlic press. Mix with the salt. Add ground coriander seeds. Mix. Dissolve in wine vinegar. Add cold water.

B. 6–8 cloves of garlic	
Salt	½–¾ cup bouillon or water

Salt the cleaned garlic and crush in a mortar or in a garlic press until a thick mass forms. Then place in a bowl. Pour the bouillon or cold water over and mix.

The sauces are served with cold dishes, with broiled or roasted turkey, chicken, fish, and lamb.

Tkemali Sauce (For meat and fish)   Georgia

2 cups damson plums   Salt
Water   1 clove garlic, crushed
2 sprigs coriander   2 sprigs dill
Hot pepper   1 sprig mint

Place washed damsons in a saucepan with just enough water to cover them, and allow to cook. When the damsons are soft and fall apart, take them off the stove and press the plums and their broth through a sieve or colander. Spice the sauce, which should be of medium consistency, with coriander, hot pepper, salt, crushed garlic, dill, and mint. Mix well.

DESSERTS

Nut Kozinak

½ cup water   ½ lb. molasses
¾ lb. powdered sugar   1½ lb. shelled walnuts, chopped
    1 tsp. vanilla

Place the water and powdered sugar in a pot and bring to a boil. Boil on a low flame for five minutes. Add molasses, and allow the syrup to continue boiling for another 3 to 4 minutes. Stir constantly. Add half the chopped walnuts. Continue cooking. After 5 to 7 minutes add the remaining nuts and cook for another 6 to 8 minutes at a temperature of 130–140° F. Empty the mixture onto a table. (A marble block, well-greased with butter, makes an excellent surface.) Allow the mixture to cool to a temperature of 80–90° (about 10 minutes). Add vanilla to the mixture. Press down the mixture into a flat block. Divide the cooled mass into several large pieces, and cut each into layers about one-half inch thick. Cut these layers into pieces (2 by 2 inches) and place on wooden boards. Cool for 45 minutes. Makes two and a half pounds. Each pound contains about thirty pieces.

Atzkhashi

1 cup honey   1–1½ cup cornmeal
1 cup water

Mix the honey and water and bring to a boil in a saucepan. Add the cornmeal gradually, stirring constantly, until a thick porridge forms. Set aside to cool. *Atzkhashi* keeps for a long time and is eaten with either milk or yogurt.

Atzkhamial (Honey Cookies)   Abkhasia

1 lb. cornmeal   1¼ cup honey

Mix the cornmeal with the honey and allow to stand for several hours. Spread out on a cookie sheet as the mixture hardens. Cut into squares and bake for 30 to 40 minutes in a slow oven. Hunters carry *atzkhamial* on long trips as it is nourishing and does not spoil. It is also used for picnics in Abkhasia.

Badam-abi-nabad (Sugar Almonds)   Azerbaijan

1 lb. powdered sugar   1 lb. shelled almonds
Water   1 tsp. vanilla
     1 tsp. butter

In an 8 to 10 quart pot add half of the sugar to a little water and warm. When the syrup comes to a boil, add the washed almonds. The temperature should be about 212° F. For the first ten minutes water evaporates, first from the water, then from the almonds. The sugar of the syrup will begin to crystallize on the surfaces of the almonds. Mix constantly with a wooden spoon. Ten minutes after the syrup has begun to boil, begin gradually adding the remaining powdered sugar every three minutes. After all of the water has evaporated, the almonds become covered with a shell of sugar—the temperature should be about 270° F.

After 20 to 25 minutes remove the almonds from the pot and dissolve the sugar remaining in the pot in water. Immerse the almonds once again. Add the vanilla. After this second boiling, the almonds should be almost completely covered with shells of melted sugar. Each almond approximately doubles in weight. The second boiling lasts for 7 or 8 minutes. Stir constantly during boiling. When ready the almonds should be emptied out onto a metal table, greased with butter, and cooled to a temperature of 50 to 60° F. Makes approximately two pounds.

BIBLIOGRAPHY

Adzhindzhal, I.A. *Iz etnografii Abkhazii (The Ethnography of Abkhasia).* Sukhumi: Alashara Publishing House, 1969.

Agrba, V.B. *Abkhazskaia poeziia i ustnoe narodnoe tvorchestvo (Abkhasian Poetry and the Oral Folk Tradition).* Tbilisi: Metsniereba Publishing House, 1971.

————. *Abkhazskaia poeziia pervykh revoliutsionnykh let i ee sviazi s fol'klorom (1917–1921) (Abkhasian Poetry in the First Years of the Revolution and Its Connection with Folklore [1917–1921]).* Sukhumi: Alashara Publishing House, 1967.

Alikishiev, R.Sh. *Dolgoletie v Dagestane (Longevity in Daghestan).* Makhachkala: Daghestan Book Publishers, 1969.

Anshba, A.A. *Voprosy poetiki abkhazskogo nartskogo eposa (Problems of Poetics in the Abkhasian Nart Epics).* Tbilisi: Metsniereba Publishing House, 1970.

Aristova, T.F. *Kurdy zakavkaz'ia (The Kurds of the Transcaucasian Region).* Moscow: Nauka Publishing House, 1966.

Armianskie narodnye skazki (Armenian Folk Tales). Erevan: Aiastan Publishing House, 1965.

Azerbaidzhanskii etnograficheskii sbornik (Azerbaijanian Ethnographic Anthology). Baku: Publishing House of the Academy of Sciences of the Azerbaijan S.S.R., 1965.

Bazian, K.A. "Problemy dolgolemiia v nagornom Karabakhe" ("Some Problems of Longevity in Nagorney, Karabakh"). *Gerontologia i Geriatria,* Yearbook, Kiev: Institut Gerontologii, 1973.

Benet, Sula. *Abkhasians: The Long-Living People of the Caucasus.* New York: Holt, Rinehart and Winston, 1974.

Butkov, P.G. *Materialy dla novoi istorii Kavkaza s 1722 po 1803 god (Material for the New History of the Caucasus 1722 to 1803),* Vol. 2. St. Petersburg: 1869.

Chebotarov, D.F. and N.N. Sachuk. "The Aged in Urbanizing Societies." Paper presented at the Ninth International Congress of Gerontologists, Kiev, 1972.

Chebotarev, D.F. and N.N. Sachuk. "Sociomedical Examination of Longevous People in the USSR." *J. Geront.,* 19: 435–439 (1964).

Darginskie skazki (Darginian Fairytales). Moscow: Vostochnaia Literatura Publishing House, 1963.

Gardanov, V.K., ed. *Kavkazskii etnograficheskii sbornik IV (Caucasian Ethnographic Collection IV).* Moscow: Nauka Publishing House, 1960.

————, **ed.** *Kul'tura i byt narodov severnogo Kavkaza (The Culture and Way of Life of the Peoples of the Northern Caucasus).* Moscow: Nauka Publishing House, 1968.

————. *Obshchestvennyi stroi adygskikh narodov (The Social Structure of the Cherkessian Peoples).* Moscow: Nauka Publishing House, 1967.

Goldstein, S. "The Biology of Aging." *N. Eng. J. Med.,* 285: 1120–1129 (1971).

Guinness Book of World Records. New York: Sterling Publishing Company, 1974, pp. 25–29.

Inal-Ipa, Sh.D. *Abkhazy (Abkhasians),* 2nd ed. Sukhumi: Alashara Publishing House, 1965.

————. *Stranitsy istoricheskoi etnografii abkhazov (Pages from the Ethnographic History of the Abkhasians).* Sukhumi: Alashara Publishing House, 1971.

————. *Ocherki po istorii braka i sem'i u abkhazov (The History of Marriage and the Family Among the Abkhasians).* Sukhumi: Abgiza Editions, 1954.

Instruktzia o poriadke proviedenia meditzinskovo obsledovania i zapolnienia karty obsledovania litz 80 let i starshe (Instruction Regarding Medical Examination and Questionnaire Given to People 80 Years Old and Over). Kiev: State Medical Press of the Ukrainian SSR, 1960.

Jarvis, D.C., M.D. *Folk Medicine.* New York: Holt, Rinehart and Winston, 1958.

Kaimarazov, G.Sh. *Ocherki istorii kul'tury narodov Dagestana (The History* *of the Culture of the Peoples of Daghestan).* Moscow: Nauka Publishing House, 1971.

Kaloev, B.A. *Osetiny (Ossetians).* Moscow: Nauka Publishing House, 1971.

Kharadze, Rusudan. *Gruzinskaia semeinaia obshchina, I–II (The Georgian Extended Family).* Tbilisi: Zaria Vostoka Publishing House, 1960.

Kindarov, B.G. "Zonalnye osobennosti zdorovia, uslovii i obraz zhizni dolgozhitelei Checheno-Ingushetii" ("Regional Peculiarities of Health Conditions and Mode of Life among the Long-Living Chechen-Ingush"). *Gerontologia i geriatria,* Yearbook, Kiev: Institut Gerontologii, 1973.

Kuznetsov, Aleksandr. *Vnizu Svanetiia (Below Is Svanetia).* Moscow: Molodaia Gvardiia Publishing House, 1971.

The Main Problems of Soviet Gerontology. Kiev: Materials for the Ninth International Congress of Gerontologists, 1972.

Maliia, E.M. *Narodnoe isobrazitel'noe iskusstvo Abkhazii (The National Folk Art of Abkhasia).* Tbilisi: Metsniereba Publishing House, 1970.

Materialy II zakavkazskoi nauchnoi konferentsii gerontologov i geriatrov (Materials from the II Transcaucasian Conference of Gerontologists and Geriatrists). Baku: Ministry of Health of Azerbaijan SSR, 1968.

McKain, Walter C. "Are They Really That Old?" *Gerontologist,* 7:70–80 (1967).

Mikava, N., ed. *Skazki i legendy gor (Fairytales and Legends of the Mountains).* Moscow: Khudozhestvennaia Literatura Publishing House, 1957.

Movchan, G.Ia. *Sotzologicheskaia Kharacteristika starogo Avarskogo Zhilishcha Kavkazskii Etnograficheskii Sbornik V (Social Characteristics of the Old Avar Homestead).* Moscow: Nauka Publishing Company, 1972.

Myers, R.J. "Economic Security in the Soviet Union." *Trans. Soc. Actuaries,* 11:723–724, 745 (1959).

———. "Further Analysis of Soviet Data on Mortality and Fertility." *Public Health Reports,* 77:177–182 (1962).

———. "Comparative Analysis of Mortality in the Soviet Union." *International Population Conference,* 2 Vols., New York, 1963, pp. 35–42.

———. "Analysis of Mortality in the Soviet Union According to 1958–59 Life Tables." *Trans. Soc. Actuaries,* 16: 309–317 (1964).

Narody Kavkaza, I–II (Peoples of the Caucasus, I–II). Moscow: The Publishing House of the Academy of Sciences of the USSR, 1960.

Ocherki istorii abkhaskoi ASSR (History of Abkhasian ASSR). Sukhumi: Abgosizdat, 1960.

Osetinskie narodnye skazki (Ossetian Folk Tales). Moscow: Khudozhestvennaia Literatura Publishing House, 1959.

Pamiatniki obychnogo prava Dagestana (Landmarks of Common Law in Daghestan). Moscow: Nauka Publishing House, 1965.

Robakidze, A.I., ed. *Kavkazskii Etnograficheskii Sbornik (Caucasian Ethnographic Collection IV)*. Tbilisi: Metsniereba Publishing House, 1972.

Rosen, S., N. Preobrazhensky, S. Khechinashvili, I. Glazunov, N. Kinshidze, and H. V. Rozen. "Epidemiologic Hearing Studies in the USSR." *Archives of Otolaryngology*, 91:424–428 (1970).

Rosenfeld, A. "The Longevity Seekers." *Saturday Review of the Sciences*, pp. 47–51, March 1973.

Saidova, M. and U. Dalgat, trans. *Avarskie skazki (Avar Fairytales)*. Moscow: Khudozhestvennaia Literatura Publishing House, 1965.

Sandrygailo, ed. *Adaty Dagestanskoi Oblasti (Customary law of Daghestan region)*. Tiflis, 1899.

Sergeeva, G. A. *Archintsy (Archinians)*. Moscow: Nauka Publishing House, 1967.

Shafiro, I.B., Ia.M. Darsaniia, I.E. Kortua, and V. R. Chikvatiia. *Dolgoletnie liudi Abkhazii (The Longevous People of Abkhasia)*. Sukhumi: The Abkhasian State Press, 1956.

Shaginian, Marietta. *Sovetskoe Zakavkazie (The Soviet Transcaucasian Region)*. Erevan: Armenian Government Publishing House, 1946.

Sichinava, G.N. *The Characteristic of the Nervous System and Psychological State of the Aged People of Abkhasia*. Sukhumi: Alashara Publishing House, 1956.

————. *On the Question of the Character and Range of Work Done by the Aged People of Abkhasia; Anthology of Papers by Physicians of Ostroumov Republican Hospital*. Sukhumi: Alashara Publishing House, 1965.

Skazaniia i legendy (Tales and Legends), trans. from the Georgian. Tbilisi: Zariia Vostoka Publishing House, 1963.

Smirnova, Ia.S. "Semeinyi byt i obshchestvennoe polozheniie abkhazskoi zhenshchiny" ("Family Life and Social Position of the Abkhasian Woman"). *Caucasian Ethnographic Collection I*. Moscow: Hauka Publishing House, 1955.

————. *Vospitanie rebenka u abkhazov (The Education of Children among the Abkhasians).* Moscow: Publishing House of the Academy of Sciences of the USSR, 1961.

————. "Vospitanie rebenka v adygskom aule v proshlom i nastoiashchem" ("The Upbringing of Children, Past and Present, in the Cherkessian Village"). *The Learned Notes of the Adygian Scientific Research Institute of Language, Literature, and History VIII.* Maikop, 1968.

Smyr, G.V. *Islam v Abkhazii i puti preodoleniia ego perezhitkov v sovremennykh usloviiakh (Islam in Abkhasia and the Means of Overcoming Its Vestiges in Contemporary Society).* Tbilisi: Metsniereba Publishing House, 1972.

Sovremennoe abkhazskoe selo (The Contemporary Abkhasian Village). Tbilisi: Metsniereba Publishing House, 1967.

Spasokukotskii, Iu.A., L. I. Barchenko, and E. D. Genis. *Dolgoletie i fiziologicheskaia starost' (Longevity and Physiological Aging).* Kiev: State Medical Press of the Ukrainian SSR, 1963.

Striagov, G.L. "Morbidity among the Elderly in Socio-Hygienic Conditions of Life." Paper presented at the Ninth International Congress of Gerontologists. Kiev, 1972.

Sulakvelidze, T.P. *Gruzinskie bliuda (Georgian Dishes).* Tbilisi: Publishing House of the Ministry of Trade of the Georgian SSR, 1959.

Sultanov, M. N. "Cholesterol, Protein Fractions and Acetyl-Neuraminal Acid in Longevous Population of the Nakhichevan ASSR." *Gerontologia i Geriatria,* Yearbook, Kiev: Institut Gerontologii, 1972.

————. *Kak prodlit nashu zhizn. (How to Lengthen Our Life).* Baku: Azerbaijan State Press, 1973.

Ter-Sarkisiants, A. E. *Sovremennaia sem'ia u armian (The Contemporary Family Among the Armenians).* Moscow: Nauka Publishing House, 1972.

Tokarev, S. A. *Etnografiia narodov SSSR (The Ethnography of the Peoples of the USSR).* Moscow: Moscow University Publishing House, 1958.

Trofimova, A.G. "Istoria Azerbaijanskoi Sem'i, Apsheron 1920–1950" ("History of the Azerbaijanian Family, Apsheron Region 1920–1950 Period"). *Caucasian Ethnographic Collection IV.* Moscow: Nauka Publishing Company, 1969.

INDEX